The AOTA Practice Guidelines Series

Occupational Therapy Practice Guidelines *for*

Home Modifications

Carol Siebert, MS, OTR/L, FAOTA
Principal
The Home Remedy
Chapel Hill (North Carolina)

Stacy Smallfield, DrOT, MSOT, OTR/L
Associate Professor
Department of Occupational Therapy
University of South Dakota
Vermillion

Susy Stark, PhD, OTR/L, FAOTA
Assistant Professor of Occupational Therapy,
*   Neurology and Social Work*
Washington University in St. Louis
St. Louis

D1245707

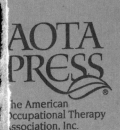

AOTA
PRESS

he American
)ccupational Therapy
ssociation, Inc.

AOTA Centennial Vision

We envision that occupational therapy is a powerful, widely recognized, science-driven, and evidence-based profession with a globally connected and diverse workforce meeting society's occupational needs.

AOTA Vision Statement

The American Occupational Therapy Association advances occupational therapy as the pre-eminent profession in promoting the health, productivity, and quality of life of individuals and society through the therapeutic application of occupation.

AOTA Mission Statement

The American Occupational Therapy Association advances the quality, availability, use, and support of occupational therapy through standard-setting, advocacy, education, and research on behalf of its members and the public.

AOTA Staff

Frederick P. Somers, *Executive Director*
Christopher M. Bluhm, *Chief Operating Officer*

Chris Davis, *Director, AOTA Press*
Ashley Hofmann, *Development/Production Editor*
Melissa Stutzbach, *Production Editor*

Rebecca Rutberg, *Director, Marketing*
Amanda Goldman, *Marketing Specialist*
Jennifer Folden, *Marketing Specialist*

The American Occupational Therapy Association, Inc.
4720 Montgomery Lane
Bethesda, MD 20814
301-652-AOTA (2682)
TDD: 800-377-8555
Fax: 301-652-7711
www.aota.org

To order: 1-877-404-AOTA (2682)

© 2014 by the American Occupational Therapy Association, Inc.
All rights reserved.
No parts of this book may be reproduced in whole or in part by any means without permission.
Printed in the United States of America.

Disclaimers

This publication is designed to provide accurate and authoritative information in regard to the subject matter covered. It is sold or distributed with the understanding that the publisher is not engaged in rendering legal, accounting, or other professional service. If legal advice or other expert assistance is required, the services of a competent professional person should be sought.
—*From the Declaration of Principles jointly adopted by the American Bar Association and a Committee of Publishers and Associations*

It is the objective of the American Occupational Therapy Association to be a forum for free expression and interchange of ideas. The opinions expressed by the contributors to this work are their own and not necessarily those of the American Occupational Therapy Association.

ISBN-13: 978-156900-357-2
Library of Congress Control Number: 2014933853

Cover design by Jennifer Folden
Composition by Maryland Composition, Laurel, MD
Printing by Automated Graphics Systems, White Plains, MD

Contents

Best Practices and Summaries of Evidence

Implications of the Evidence for Occupational Therapy Research, Education, and Clinical Practice

Appendixes

References

Subject Index

Citation Index

Figures, Exhibits, Tables, and Boxes

Acknowledgments

The series editor for this Practice Guideline is

Deborah Lieberman, MHSA, OTR/L, FAOTA
Director, Evidence-Based Practice
Staff Liaison to the Commission on Practice
American Occupational Therapy Association
Bethesda, MD

The issue editor for this Practice Guideline is

Marian Arbesman, PhD, OTR/L
President, ArbesIdeas, Inc.
Consultant, AOTA Evidence-Based Practice Project
Clinical Assistant Professor, Department of
    Rehabilitation Science
State University of New York at Buffalo

The authors acknowledge the following individuals
for their contributions to the evidence-based literature review:

Susy Stark, PhD, OTR/L, FAOTA
Marian Keglovits, OTD/S
Graduate students in the lab of Susy Stark, PhD,
    OTR/L, FAOTA

The authors acknowledge and thank the following
individuals for their participation in the content
review and development of this publication:

Susan Bachner, MA, OTR/L, FAOTA, SCEM,
    CEAC, CAPS
Carla A. Chase, EdD, OTR/L
Richard C. Duncan, MRP
Tiffanie Kinney
Marnie Renda, MEd, OTR/L, CAPS, ECHM
Dory Sabata, OTD, OTR/L, SCEM
Christina A. Metzler
Karen Smith, OT/L, CAPS
V. Judith Thomas, MGA
Madalene Palmer

Note. The authors of this Practice Guideline have
signed a Conflict of Interest statement indicating
that they have no conflicts that would bear on this
work.

Introduction

Purpose and Use of This Publication

Practice guidelines have been widely developed in response to the health care reform movement in the United States. Such guidelines can be useful tools for improving the quality of health care, enhancing consumer satisfaction, promoting appropriate use of services, and reducing costs. The American Occupational Therapy Association (AOTA), which represents nearly 150,000 occupational therapists, occupational therapy assistants (see Appendix A), and students of occupational therapy, is committed to providing information through relevant practice guidelines and other resources to support decision making that promotes a high-quality health care system that is affordable and accessible to all. Readers should also refer to home modification information in the Productive Aging section of AOTA's website.

Using an evidence-based perspective and key concepts from the *Occupational Therapy Practice Framework: Domain and Process* (3rd ed., AOTA, 2014), this guideline provides an overview of the occupational therapy process for providing home modification interventions. It defines the occupational therapy domain and process and interventions that occur within the boundaries of acceptable practice. This guideline does not discuss all possible methods of care, and although it does recommend some specific methods of care, occupational therapists make a professional determination regarding the appropriateness of a given intervention in light of a specific person's circumstances and needs as

well as the evidence available to support the intervention. The final decision about modifications is made in conjunction with the client.

It is the intention of AOTA, through this publication, to help occupational therapists and occupational therapy assistants, as well as those who manage, reimburse, or set policy regarding occupational therapy services, understand the contribution of occupational therapy for home modification interventions. This guideline can also serve as a reference for health care professionals, health care facility managers, education and health care regulators, third-party payers, and managed care organizations. Selected diagnostic and billing code information for evaluations and interventions is provided in Appendix B.

This document may be used in any of the following ways:
- To assist occupational therapists and occupational therapy assistants in communicating about their services to external audiences;
- To assist community partners, physicians, other health care practitioners, case managers, families and caregivers, and health care facility managers in determining whether referral for occupational therapy services would be appropriate;
- To assist third-party payers in determining the medical necessity for occupational therapy;
- To assist legislators, third-party payers, and administrators in understanding the professional education, training, and skills of occupational therapists and occupational therapy assistants;
- To assist health and education planning teams in determining the need for occupational therapy;

- To assist program developers, administrators, legislators, and third-party payers in understanding the scope of occupational therapy services;
- To assist program evaluators and policy analysts in this practice area in determining outcome measures for analyzing the effectiveness of occupational therapy intervention;
- To assist policy, education, and health care benefit analysts in understanding the appropriateness of occupational therapy services for home modifications;
- To assist policymakers, legislators, and organizations in understanding the contribution occupational therapy can make to program development and health care reform for home modifications;
- To assist occupational therapy educators in designing appropriate curricula that incorporate the role of occupational therapy in the area of home modifications; and
- To assist consumers of occupational therapy services to better understand the depth and breadth of knowledge and services available in the area of home modifications.

The introduction to this guideline continues with a brief discussion of the domain and process of occupational therapy. This discussion is followed by a detailed description of the occupational therapy process for home modifications, including a summary of evidence from the literature regarding best practices. Embedded within these descriptions are summaries of the results of a systematic review of evidence from the scientific literature regarding best practices in occupational therapy intervention for home modifications. Finally, appendixes contain the methodology and evidence tables for the review (see Appendixes C and D, respectively) and guide-lines related to using *CPT*[TM] codes for billing (see Appendix B).

Domain and Process of Occupational Therapy

Occupational therapy practitioners' expertise lies in their knowledge of occupation and of how engaging in occupations can be used to support health and participation in home, school, the workplace, and community life.

In 2013, the AOTA Representative Assembly adopted the *Occupational Therapy Practice Framework: Domain and Process* (3rd ed.; AOTA, 2014). Informed by the first and second editions of the *Occupational Therapy Practice Framework: Domain and Process* (AOTA, 2002, 2008), the previous *Uniform Terminology for Occupational Therapy* (AOTA, 1989, 1994), and the World Health Organization's (2001) *International Classification of Functioning, Disability and Health,* the *Framework* outlines the profession's domain and the process of service delivery within this domain.

Domain

A profession's *domain* articulates its sphere of knowledge, societal contribution, and intellectual or scientific activity. The occupational therapy profession's domain centers on helping others participate in daily life activities. The broad term that the profession uses to describe daily life activities is *occupation*. As outlined in the *Framework,* occupational therapists and occupational therapy assistants[1] work collaboratively with people, groups, and populations (clients) to engage in everyday activities or occupations that they want and need to do in a manner that supports health and participation (see Figure 1).

---

[1]*Occupational therapists* are responsible for all aspects of occupational therapy service delivery and are accountable for the safety and effectiveness of the occupational therapy service delivery process. *Occupational therapy assistants* deliver occupational therapy services under the supervision of and in partnership with an occupational therapist (AOTA, 2009).

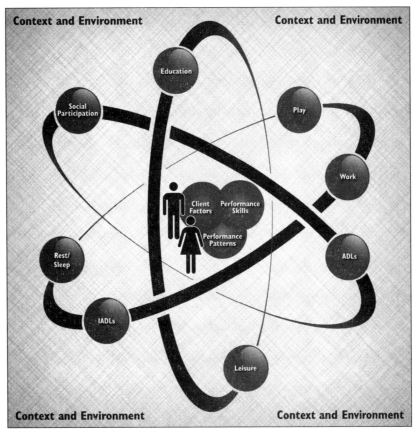

Figure 1. Occupational therapy's domain.

Note. ADLs = activities of daily living; IADLs = instrumental activities of daily living.
Source. Occupational Therapy Practice Framework: Domain and Process (3rd ed., p. S5), by
American Occupational Therapy Association, 2014, *American Journal of Occupational Therapy,*
68(Suppl. 1), S1–S48. Used with permission.

Using occupational engagement as both the desired outcome of intervention and the intervention itself, occupational therapy practitioners[2] are skilled at viewing the subjective and objective aspects of performance and understanding occupation simultaneously from this dual, yet holistic, perspective. The overarching statement "achieving health, well-being, and participation in life through engagement in occupation" (AOTA, 2014, p. S2) circumscribes the profession's domain and emphasizes the important ways that environmental and life circumstances influence the manner in which people carry out their occupations. Key aspects of the domain of occupational therapy are defined in Exhibit 1.

Process

A wide range of professionals use the process of evaluating, intervening, and targeting outcomes

---

[2]When the term *occupational therapy practitioner* is used in this document, it refers to both occupational therapists and occupational therapy assistants (AOTA, 2006).

OCCUPATIONS	CLIENT FACTORS	PERFORMANCE SKILLS	PERFORMANCE PATTERNS	CONTEXTS AND ENVIRONMENTS
Activities of daily living (ADLs)*	Values, beliefs, and spirituality	Motor skills	Habits	Cultural
Instrumental activities of daily living (IADLs)	Body functions	Process skills	Routines	Personal
	Body structures	Social interaction skills	Rituals	Physical
Rest and sleep			Roles	Social
Education				Temporal
Work				Virtual
Play				
Leisure				
Social participation				
*Also referred to as *basic activities of daily living (BADLs)* or *personal activities of daily living (PADLs)*.				

Exhibit 1. Aspects of the domain of occupational therapy.

Note. All aspects of the domain transact to support engagement, participation, and health. This exhibit does not imply a hierarchy.
Source. Occupational Therapy Practice Framework: Domain and Process (3rd ed., p. S4), by American Occupational Therapy Association, 2014, *American Journal of Occupational Therapy, 68*(Suppl. 1), S1–S48. Used with permission.

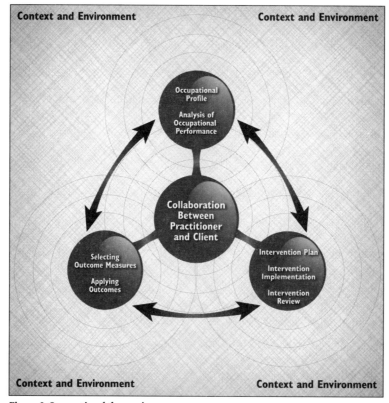

Figure 2. Occupational therapy's process.

Source. Occupational Therapy Practice Framework: Domain and Process (3rd ed., p. S10), by American Occupational Therapy Association, 2014, *American Journal of Occupational Therapy, 68*(Suppl. 1), S1–S48. Used with permission.

outlined in the *Framework*. Occupational therapy's application of this process is made unique, however, by its focus on occupation (see Figure 2). The process of occupational therapy service delivery typically begins with the *occupational profile*, an assessment of the client's occupational needs, problems, and concerns, and the *analysis of occupational performance*, which includes the skills, patterns, contexts and environments, activity demands, and client factors that contribute to or impede the client's satisfaction with his or her ability to engage in valued daily life activities. Therapists then plan and implement intervention using a variety of approaches and methods in which occupation is both the means and the ends (Trombly, 1995).

Occupational therapists continually assess the effectiveness of the intervention and the client's progress toward targeted outcomes. The intervention review informs decisions to continue or discontinue intervention and to make referrals to other agencies or professionals.

Overview of Occupational Therapy for Home Modifications

Home modifications are generally provided to improve functional performance, reduce home hazards to prevent falls or other injuries, and reduce the demands on caregivers. Home modifications provided by occupational therapists involve a multistep process, including

1. A comprehensive evaluation of personal and environmental factors and daily activities;
2. The development of an intervention plan to resolve the incompatibilities between the person and the environment;
3. The facilitation of obtaining or installing the modifications; and
4. Training in the use of the modifications.

The need for home modifications arises when the features of the environment pose challenges or demands that are incompatible with an occupant's ability to address the challenges or demands safely and effectively. Such incompatibility may be the result of impairment, such as those associated with a health condition or changes in abilities associated with aging. Incompatibility often results in limitations in the person's ability to participate in the home and community.

Modifications include a set of strategies to compensate for impairments and improve performance of daily activities. Strategies can include medical equipment (e.g., tub bench), universally designed products (e.g., easy-to-grip utensils), architectural modifications (e.g., ramp), major home renovations (e.g., roll-in shower), or learning a strategy to use the environment in a different way (e.g., turn on the light before walking down stairs). All occupational therapists are qualified to conduct home assessments and deliver home modification interventions, although some occupational therapists may have advanced practice skills for complex home modification interventions.

The outcome of home modifications provided by occupational therapists is enhanced occupational performance. The process may occur with more than one occupational therapy practitioner at different stages along the health care continuum.

Home modifications support engagement and participation (in the home and in the community). This guideline addresses home modifications as an intervention to use when a person's abilities are incompatible with environmental demands. That intervention includes identifying, developing, implementing, and training in the use of home modifications.

Home modifications vary in focus and may be part of a single-component intervention (home modifications only) or a multicomponent intervention (home modifications as part of a comprehensive intervention package). Comprehensive, evidence-based interventions include an evaluation of personal abilities and environmental factors using psychometrically sound assessments in the home as well as adequate follow-up and support (Clemson, Mackenzie, Ballinger, Close, & Cumming, 2008). Home modification interventions that incorporate these essential ingredients result in decreased falls and increased function for community-dwelling adults (Brunnström, Sörensen, Alsterstad, & Sjöstrand, 2004; Campbell et al., 2005; Davison, Bond, Dawson, Steen, & Kenny, 2005; Gitlin et al., 2006; La Grow, Robertson, Campbell, Clarke, &

Kerse, 2006; Stark, Landsbaum, Palmer, Somerville, & Morris, 2009). Comprehensive environmental interventions improve participation for adults in the home and the community (Clemson et al., 2008).

The following sections provide an overview of occupational therapy practice and home modifications. Nuances of this area of service delivery are described, including differences from other areas of occupational therapy practice.

Service Delivery Contexts

Home modifications are appropriate for people of all ages to improve function, increase safety, decrease caregiver burden, and increase life participation. Home modifications are appropriate for people with a broad range of health conditions or people who are at risk of developing health conditions because of the presence of barriers in the home. Home modifications are an appropriate intervention for people with impairments in a broad range of functional areas that include behavioral, cognitive, and physical functioning. Home modifications can also support people with acute temporary to chronic progressive disease processes.

Home modifications are also important as a method of prevention—to remove home hazards to prevent falls or to improve the person's ability to perform daily activities as a means to prevent disability. Home modifications may be addressed in a variety of service delivery contexts. In situations in which a client has experienced a sudden change in abilities, as in the case of an acute health condition, the need for or initial planning of home modifications may begin in a hospital, rehabilitation, or home health care setting. Incompatibilities may also develop gradually, as in situations in which a client's abilities change as a result of a chronic progressive condition or in association with the aging process. In these circumstances, the client may want to resolve these incompatibilities through the services of an outpatient setting, home health agency, or community-based practice.

Interprofessional Team Involvement

Occupational therapy practitioners practicing in home modifications are most commonly part of an interprofessional home modifications team. The composition of this team varies depending on the practice circumstances and the modification to be completed. Members of the interprofessional team always include the client and may include contractors; tradespeople including plumbers, electricians, and carpenters; architects; interior designers; rehabilitation engineers; handypersons; and volunteers from home repair or community service organizations (see Table 1 for home modification team members and their roles). The team may include other health professionals, such as nurses, physical therapists, and social workers. Team members may also provide overall coordination of services for the client or coordinate both services and funding. These team members may include case managers, life care planners, project coordinators, and representatives from a funding agency.

The Home as a Context for Practice

Home modification practice occurs in a specific and unique context: the client's home. The context is the venue for practice, but it is also the medium for intervention. These circumstances demand an appreciation of the meaning of home to the client, an understanding of how practicing in the home alters the practitioner–client dynamic, and an appreciation of the meaning of home to the client.

Meaning of *Home*

For the client, *home* is more than a physical structure. Home consists of both the physical space and the memories, objects, and meanings associated with the structure by those who dwell in it. Intimate

Table 1. Interprofessional Home Modification Team Member Roles

Team Member	Role on the Home Modification Team
Client	• Participates in the evaluation of performance of daily activities at home. • Reviews the range of intervention options available and selects preferred home modification for implementation. • Receives training in the use of home modification interventions after installation.
Family members	• Provide additional input for changes, especially in areas of shared space. • Understand the roles and occupations of the family members currently living in the home. • May receive training in the use of home modification interventions after installation.
Occupational therapist	• Evaluates the client's performance of occupations in the home. • Identifies supports and hindrances to occupational performance in the home. • Identifies a range of options for removing hindrances and maximizing occupational performance in collaboration with team members. • Communicates recommendations to the interprofessional team. • Implements intervention options in collaboration with team members. • Provides follow-up education and training to the client and family members to integrate the home modifications into daily performance patterns.
Contractors	• Understand building construction. • Provide guidance as to modification possibilities. • Estimate the cost of home modifications. • Install the identified home renovations. • Hire and supervise any identified subcontractors as appropriate (i.e., plumbing, electrical). • Understand local building codes. • Coordinate complex teams of building professionals.
Interior designers	• Assist with the design of the interior space, including lighting, acoustics, organization, storage, scale, accommodation of special needs, and compliance with local building codes. • Collaborate with the home modification team to identify potential intervention options.
Architect	• Designs the physical layout of the space with consideration of aesthetics, space use, and other architectural elements. • Prepares plans needed to obtain building permit. • Understands local building codes and regulations. • Coordinates complex teams of building professionals, which may include interior designers, contractors, engineers, and others.

and ongoing interaction with a physical context transforms a space into a place (Tuan, 1977). Identification with the home is a dynamic transaction (Cooper Marcus, 1997). For people who have lived in a home for many decades, the home is an extension of the self (Rowles, 1991, 2000, 2008). Home modifications may be a person's first tangible acknowledgment that performance is changing or has changed.

Although *home modifications* refers to modifications of the home's physical environment, such modifications may effect a change for the client that goes beyond how the client physically interacts with the features of the home or the objects in it. Even apparently minor changes such as rearranging furniture or removing apparent clutter may produce more than a minor alteration in the client's sense of home and being at home (Hasselkus, 2011). The meaning of home and of specific spaces and objects must be discerned, respected, and, whenever possible, maintained as modifications are planned and implemented. Attention to aesthetics is an important consideration for the client and interprofessional intervention team.

Family Members

Family members or other occupants of the home have a stake in the home modifications and may be affected by them. Some home modifications may be desired specifically for their impact on a family member. Changes to the home environment may also have an impact on the meaning of home for occupants other than the identified client. Family members have a dual role in home modifications: (1) as clients who will benefit or be affected by the interventions and (2) as members of the team who may participate in planning or implementing the modifications.

In situations in which home modifications are sought to relieve the burden or risk associated with caregiving, the caregiver benefits from the modifi-cations, as does the identified client. Both parties will be involved in the process of evaluation and identification of appropriate modifications so that the modifications are compatible with the abilities and needs of both client and caregiver.

The home has meaning for all the occupants of the home, and meanings may differ for each person. Some modifications affect the use of the home or activities in the home for the client only. However, if modifications are proposed in any area of the home that is used by occupants other than the client, other occupants' abilities and needs must be considered. Failure to take these issues into consideration may result in opposition to the modifica-tions or may produce unanticipated incompatibili-ties for other members of the household.

Occupational Therapy Process for Home Modifications

Referral

The need for home modifications may be precipitated by a change in a person's ability, a change in the home environment, a change in what the client needs or wants to do, or a combination of these factors. Home modifications may also be used as a prevention strategy (e.g., fall risk reduction).

Just as need for home modifications may arise from a variety of circumstances, referrals for home modifications may arise in a variety of ways. In some cases, home modification may be the purpose of a referral (or self-referral) for occupational therapy services. In others, addressing home modifications may be part of a broader referral for occupational therapy services. For example, a person seeking home modifications to prevent falls may be referred by his or her geriatrician for a home hazard removal intervention by occupational therapists. In contrast, occupational therapy may be provided when a person is referred for home health care. Home modifications may be one of multiple interventions identified by occupational therapists.

More often, the need for home modifications may not be apparent to the person experiencing performance difficulties. This situation most commonly occurs when a person experiences an abrupt change in abilities. In these situations, the person may be referred for occupational therapy to restore abilities or to learn compensatory strategies. As the client receives services directed toward skills and activities, occupational therapists may also identify the need to modify the environment to restore compatibility. The need for home modifications may be identified as part of discharge planning from an inpatient facility or as an aspect of outpatient or home health services (Schawe & Crist, 2013).

At other times, a person's abilities change gradually or are anticipated to change or decline. This change may be associated with a chronic progressive health condition or with aging. The person may recognize or anticipate incompatibilities and initiate a referral for home modifications, or the person may seek occupational therapy services for rehabilitation or compensation and, in the process, the need for home modification is also identified.

Referrals may also come from other professionals or organizations that serve people experiencing incompatibilities among abilities, activities, and the home environment. They include, but are not limited to, service and advocacy organizations serving people with specific health conditions, independent living centers or programs, area agencies on aging, service organizations offering housing repair or renovation services, contractors, vocational rehabilitation services, Medicaid waiver programs, attorneys, case managers, and life care planners (Schawe & Crist, 2013).

Evaluation

Occupational therapists perform evaluations in collaboration with the client and target information specific to the desired outcomes such as reducing caregiver burden or reducing fall risk. The two elements of the occupational therapy evaluation are (1) the occupational profile and (2) the analysis of occupational performance (AOTA, 2014).

Occupational therapists working in home modifications may use standardized and nonstandardized assessments. Occupational therapists should validate clinical observations with data from standardized assessments. Consistent use of standardized assessments across the continuum of care during the disease process enhances continuity of care and allows for retrospective analysis of client outcomes, contributing to the evidence supporting practice. Table 2 provides a brief overview of selected assessments that may be used for evaluation of the home environment.

Occupational Profile

The purpose of the occupational profile is to determine who the client or clients are, identify their needs or concerns, and ascertain how these concerns affect engagement in occupational performance. Information for the occupational profile is gathered through formal and informal interviews with the client and significant others. Formal assessments may include the Canadian Occupational Performance Measure (COPM; Law et al., 2005) or the Activity Card Sort (Baum & Edwards, 2008). Conversations with the client help occupational therapists gain perspective on how the client spends his or her time; what activities the client wants or needs to do; and how the environment in which the client lives, works, and plays supports or hinders occupational engagement.

The occupational profile provides occupational therapists with the opportunity to understand the background details of a client's life that are not necessarily part of a health condition but could play an important role in the outcome of the intervention. Some of these details can greatly influence adherence and acceptance of home modifications (Stark, Somerville, & Keglovits, 2013). Occupational therapists who do not consider these personal factors are more likely to have clients who abandon the home modifications. Stark et al. (2013) found that personal factors important to understand for

successful home modifications include a client's readiness for change (Tabbarah, Silverstein, & Seeman, 2000), personality traits (Costa & McCrae, 1992), disease status (temporary, chronic, progressive), tolerance for personal assistance, ability to operate and maintain modifications, compliance with instructions to maintain safety, concern for aesthetics, health literacy, financial resources, social support, home ownership, coresidents (including pets), and plan for future moves. Although not formally assessed, these personal factors will strongly influence the development of an intervention plan and should be ascertained during the occupational profile.

Developing the occupational profile involves the following steps:
- Identify the client or clients. During the home modification process, multiple clients may be involved. For example, the recipient of the intervention might be the person with a disabling condition or the person's caregiver. Multiple clients may provide information for the occupational profile.
- Determine why the client is seeking services. Through interviews or assessment, occupational therapists assist the client in identifying current concerns relative to engaging in occupations and daily life activities. The client's ability to identify and establish goals is essential to the home modifications process.
- Identify the occupations in which the client feels successful and the barriers that affect his or her success.
- Identify aspects of the environment or context that the client perceives as supporting engagement in desired occupations and aspects that are inhibiting engagement.
- Discuss significant aspects of the client's occupational history (e.g., life experiences). Significant aspects may include medical interventions, employment history, vocational preferences, occupational roles, interests, and previous patterns of engagement in occupations that

Table 2. Selected Occupational Therapy Home Modification Assessments

Assessment	Description
Craig Hospital Inventory of Environmental Factors (CHIEF) and CHIEF Short Form (Harrison-Felix, 2001)	A general assessment of environmental barriers in the areas of accessibility, accommodation, resources, social support, and equality. The Long Form contains 25 items, and the Short Form contains 12 items. It is not specific to the home environment.
Housing Enabler (Iwarsson & Slaug, 2001)	A comprehensive audit tool based on environmental press theory. It includes 15 possible functional limitations of the client and 188 possible environmental barriers to identify potential problem areas on the basis of the interaction between them. The client need not be present when conducting the audit.
Comprehensive Assessment and Solution Process for Aging Adults (CASPAR; Sanford, Pynoos, Tejral, & Browne, 2001)	A home assessment tool designed to identify client priorities, the client's ability to participate in daily activities in the home, and the layout and design of the home. It was designed to be used by occupational therapists without the requirement of being onsite to complete the evaluation.
Home Falls and Accidents Screening Tool (HOME FAST; MacKenzie, Byles, & Higginbotham, 2000)	A home audit tool that contains yes–no questions for identifying hazards in the home. The client need not be present when conducting the audit.
In-Home Occupational Performance Evaluation (I–HOPE; Stark, Somerville, & Morris, 2010)	An assessment of occupational performance in the home environment. It consists of 44 activities rated on a 5-point scale. It provides scores for activity participation, activity performance, satisfaction with performance, and severity of environmental barriers.
Lifease (Christenson, 1991) and Buildease (Christenson, 2006)	Computer-based home assessment and modification tools that create a customized checklist on the basis of a person's disability. A database of potential solutions and products for identified problem areas is also included.
Safety Assessment of Function and the Environment for Rehabilitation–Health Outcome Measurement Evaluation, Version 3 (SAFER–HOME v.3; Chiu et al., 2006)	An assessment of safety in the home environment for older adults and people with disabilities. It is a checklist of 75 questions divided into 12 categories of ADLs and IADLs, each rated on problem severity.
Westmead Home Safety Assessment (WeHSA; Clemson, 1997)	A clinical and research assessment tool for identifying hazards in the home. It consists of a 72-section checklist grouped by home category and was designed to assist in fall prevention.
Home Environment Assessment Protocol (HEAP; Gitlin et al., 2002)	A clinical and research assessment tool developed to identify safety hazards in the home for people with dementia and based on environmental press theory. It includes 192 items in 8 areas of the home. Safety hazards are identified as trip and fall hazards, electrical issues, or access to dangerous items.

Note. ADLs = activities of daily living; IADLs = instrumental activities of daily living.

provide meaning to the client's life. It is also important to explore the meaning of home and the various areas of the home.

- Discuss the client's values and interests. Identify the client's daily life roles. Determine the client's patterns of engagement in occupations and how they have changed over time.

- Determine the client's priorities and desired outcomes in relation to occupational performance, prevention, health and wellness, quality of life, participation, role competence, well-being, and occupational justice. Throughout the rehabilitative process, the occupational therapist and client will discuss and prioritize goals so that the therapist's evaluation and interventions will match the client's desired outcomes. At times, occupational therapists may need to refer clients to additional professionals or resources to achieve successful outcomes. It is also important to understand what changes in the home clients are willing to make to achieve these goals and the types of resources, both financial and personal, available to implement them.

Analysis of Occupational Performance

Occupational therapists uses information from the occupational profile to focus on the specific areas of occupation in relationship to the context and environment in which the client will live and function.

When occupational therapists evaluate occupational performance, the following steps are generally included:

- Observe the client as he or she performs the occupations in the natural or least restrictive environment (when possible), and note the effectiveness of the client's performance skills (e.g., motor skills, process skills, and social interaction skills and performance patterns, such as habits, routines, rituals, roles).
- Select specific evaluation tools and methods that will identify and measure the factors related to the specific aspects of the domain of practice that may be influencing the client's performance. These factors include evaluation of body structures and functions, activity performance, and community participation.
- Interpret the evaluation data to identify what supports or hinders performance.
- Develop or refine a hypothesis regarding the client's performance (i.e., identify underlying impairments or performance skill limitations that may be influencing occupational performance in multiple areas, such as a mismatch

between the client's skills and the home environment affecting morning self-care, home management tasks, functional mobility, and leisure activities).
- Develop goals in collaboration with the client and possibly the family that address the client's desired outcomes.
- Identify potential intervention approaches, guided by best practice and the evidence, and discuss them with the client, family, or both.
- Document the evaluation process and communicate the results to the appropriate team members and community agencies.

Areas of Occupation

Evaluation of the home environment includes an assessment of the client's ability to perform his or her regular occupations in that setting. It provides a baseline status of occupational performance in the natural home environment rather than in an artificial clinical setting (Stark, Somerville, & Russell-Thomas, 2011). Therefore, occupational therapy practitioners can use the information gathered at baseline to determine the effectiveness of the home modification strategies that were implemented.

The most commonly assessed occupations for adults during a home modification evaluation include activities of daily living (ADLs), instrumental activities of daily living (IADLs), rest and sleep, leisure, and social participation. The areas of work, education, and play should also be included in a home evaluation if relevant for the client, because many clients participating in a home modification evaluation either are retired or work out of the home.

The COPM (Law et al., 2005) is a formal assessment tool that can be used to determine the areas of most importance to the client in home modification evaluation. The COPM is a semistructured interview that occupational therapy practitioners can use to identify the client's meaningful but difficult-to-perform occupations. The results of this assessment tool can serve as a guide to home modification, because occupational therapy practitioners can introduce modifications to enhance the occupation–environment fit for these identified occupations.

Occupational therapy practitioners often integrate home modification into a variety of service delivery contexts. These contexts may include the hospital (e.g., acute care setting, intensive inpatient rehabilitation program), postacute rehabilitation as experienced in a short-term stay in a skilled nursing facility or swing-bed unit, home health care, or outpatient rehabilitation program. Because of this variation in service delivery contexts, variation may occur in the standardized assessment tools that are associated with home modification practice. Occupational therapists may often use formal standardized assessments in the primary service delivery context before the home evaluation. Therefore, occupational therapists can compare the information gathered using a standardized assessment of occupation, which is often performed in the artificial context of an institutional setting, with the information gathered by observation of occupational performance in the natural home environment.

Another occupation that occupational therapists should assess during a home modification evaluation is sleep and rest. In particular, a client's ability to prepare for sleep, including donning sleep garments, performing routine bedtime activities, transferring into and out of bed, and nighttime toileting, is critical for living safely and independently at home. Occupational therapists assessing occupations of sleep and rest observe the client perform any of the tasks that make up the bedtime or resting routine to analyze the fit between the client's skill and ability to perform the tasks in the home environment.

Similarly, occupational therapists assess the education, work, play, leisure, and social participation areas of occupation largely by informal observation rather than with a standardized assessment tool. Occupational therapists assessing these areas would want to work with the client to identify the locations in the home in which homework, class activities, leisure activities, socializing, or work tasks are most often completed and then observe the client performing those tasks. These activities might include observing the client performing paper-and-pencil homework assignments; studying from a textbook; or navigating a virtual classroom setting using a desktop, laptop, or tablet computer. Assessment of leisure and social participation may include observation of a wide variety of activities including, but not limited to, functional mobility and transfers in common areas of the home or accessing the telephone or television. Observation of work tasks may include computer-related tasks but may also include work tasks associated with other home business such as the creation of arts and crafts or other handiwork. Occupational therapists would record any hindrances the client might have performing those activities in the home environment to inform the intervention planning process.

Because observation of occupational performance in the home environment is the most common way to determine which attributes of the built environment are hindering performance (Stark et al., 2011), several authors have designed assessments that specifically measure the interaction between the person and the home environment either in person (Chiu et al., 2006; Stark, Somerville, & Morris, 2010) or remotely (Hoenig et al., 2006). These assessments can assist in objectively describing the impact of the environment on performance and in determining strategies to reduce barriers that may be present. Two examples are briefly described here (see also Table 2 for further information about common occupational therapy home modification assessments).

One assessment that focuses on the fit between the client and his or her environment is the In-Home Occupational Therapy Evaluation (I–HOPE; Stark et al., 2010), which measures performance difficulties the client has in the home environment on the basis of tasks that have been identified as essential for aging in place (Stark et al., 2010). Occupational therapists observe the performance of problematic activities to identify the barriers that hinder successful performance. The I–HOPE was also designed to consider the client's satisfaction with his or her performance of the activity. Occupational therapists can use the I–HOPE as a premeasure and a postmeasure of performance so that the change in performance on the basis of a home modification intervention can be documented (Stark et al., 2010).

Another occupational therapy assessment of the fit between the person and the home environment is the Safety Assessment of Function and the Environment for Rehabilitation–Health Outcome and Measurement Evaluation, version 3 (SAFER–HOME v.3; Chiu et al., 2006). The SAFER–HOME v.3 contains 74 task performance items, each rated on a 4-point scale ranging from 0 = *no identified problem* to 3 = *severe problem* (Chiu et al., 2006). It is both a clinical measure of the client's ability to perform occupations in the home environment and an outcome measure to evaluate the effectiveness of the intervention strategies that the occupational therapy practitioner used to address the identified problem areas (Chiu et al., 2006).

Performance Skills

The evaluation of the person–home environment fit includes assessing overt and subtle factors that may affect performance. *Performance skills* are goal-directed actions that are observable as small units of engagement in daily life occupations. They are learned and developed over time and are situated in specific contexts and environments (Fisher & Griswold, 2014). Fisher and Griswold (2014) categorized performance skills as motor skills, process skills, and social interaction skills. Clients receiving a home modification evaluation may present with deficits in one or many of these performance skills. Occupational therapists may assess these skills using standardized assessments or informal observation of occupational performance.

Occupational therapists can use the Assessment of Motor and Process Skills (AMPS; Fisher, 1995) and the Performance Assessment of Self-Care Skills (PASS; Rogers & Holm, 1994) to evaluate performance skills. Practitioners may select from a variety of tasks that are relevant to the specific client's impaired performance area (Fisher, 1995; Rogers & Holm, 1994). Both tools determine quality of performance rather than the sole outcome of performance (Rogers & Holm, 1994). The PASS also includes a rating of safety (Rogers & Holm, 1994).

Clients receiving a home modification evaluation often have impaired motor skills as a result of their underlying medical condition. It is imperative for occupational therapists to observe the client's motor skills to understand how these impairments affect the client's safety and independence in the home setting. Many opportunities are available to observe motor and process skills while the client is performing occupations of choice. For example, occupational therapists can observe motor and process skills when the client sequences the motor task of transferring to the toilet from a wheelchair or walker, bends or reaches to retrieve food from the refrigerator, or sequences the steps of a carrying out a cooking task in the kitchen using a walker. Additional opportunities to assess motor and process skills may include observing the client navigate steps into the home or maintain balance while transferring laundry from the washer to the dryer. The information gleaned through careful observation of motor and process skills is critical to the overall home modification evaluation and intervention planning process because determining whether these skills are intact, absent, or impaired will influence the intervention strategies that occupational therapists recommend.

Similarly, process skills are critical to living safely in the home environment because the client uses these skills to identify, locate, and respond to information present in the environment. A mismatch between the client and the home environment in the area of processing sensory information will require skilled intervention strategies to ensure that the client is safe. Specifically, occupational therapists will want to observe the client's ability to hear and react to auditory alerts such as the smoke detector, oven timer, telephone, or doorbell. Likewise, occupational therapists should also observe the visual identification of important information, such as identifying spoiled food in the refrigerator or reacting appropriately to food as it is cooking. Occupational therapists will also want to observe occupations that require the use of the tactile and proprioceptive senses, such as feeling for grab bars or testing for the appropriate water temperature. It is important for occupational therapists to identify any skill deficits to recommend necessary accommodations.

Process skills are essential to the performance of occupation (AOTA, 2014). The observable elements of process skills include the actions that demonstrate the pacing, attending, sequencing, initiating, gathering, terminating, and organizing involved in performing daily occupations (AOTA, 2014). Impairments in process skills can have a significant impact on the client's ability to perform necessary occupations; therefore, they are important to observe and record during the home modification evaluation. Process skills can be observed when the client chooses appropriate clothing items for getting dressed, sequences the steps of a cooking task appropriately, identifies solutions to a problem, or manages multiple household tasks at the same time, to name a few.

A client's social interaction skills may be affected when he or she experiences a medical condition or disability. For example, emotional lability can occur after a stroke, and adjustment to a new disability or loss of function naturally affects a person's emotional well-being. Therefore, observing social interaction skills as part of the overall home modification evaluation is critical to the success of the evaluation and resulting intervention strategies. Although natural opportunities to observe the client's emotional status throughout the home modification evaluation occur simply by noting whether the client is displaying appropriate emotions, specific behaviors may also be observed, such as when a client displays fear before a tub transfer or persists in attempting to complete a difficult task.

Finally, social interaction skills are important for effective performance of occupations in the home environment both when the client lives with others and when the client lives independently. Effective social interaction skills can include answering questions and taking turns in conversation with either a family member or a service provider, making appropriate eye contact and gestures when carrying on a conversation, or acknowledging the receipt of information. Effective social interaction skills can be especially critical when the client lives alone because caregivers who live at a distance may rely on communication to ensure the client's health and safety. When social interaction skills are impaired because of a medical or other disabling condition, home modification intervention can include strategies to assist with addressing this deficit area. Therefore, including these performance skills as part of the overall home modification evaluation is important.

Client Factors

Client factors include values, beliefs, and spirituality; body functions; and body structures that affect the client's occupational performance. Client factors are not the likely target of home modification intervention; rather, they are an important component of developing a successful intervention plan for home modifications. Most home modifications are provided using a competence–press framework that acknowledges that compensation for functional limitations can be achieved by providing environmental support (or reducing environmental barriers). A task analysis (Watson & Wilson, 2003) is conducted to determine the barriers present in the home relative to the limitations in body functions and structures. A clear understanding of the limitations in client factors is essential for this process.

Table 3. Sample Measurement Model for Use With Clients Wanting to Age in Place

Personal Factors	Instrument	Reference
Strength	Manual Muscle Testing	Hislop & Montgomery (2007)
Visual acuity	Near acuity, distance acuity	Warren (1998)
Range of motion	Goniometer	Whelan (2014)
Stages of change	Stages of Change Questionnaire	Prochaska & Velicer (1997)
Mobility	Get Up and Go Test	Mathias, Nayak, & Isaacs (1986)
Cognition	Short Blessed Memory Test	Katzman et al. (1983)
Depression	Geriatric Depression Scale, Short Form	Sheikh & Yesavage (1986)
Comorbid conditions	Charlson Comorbidity Index	Charlson, Pompei, Ales, & MacKenzie (1987)
Health-related quality of life	Short Form–36	Ware & Sherbourne (1992)

Standardized assessments can be used to screen client factors (see Table 3). These factors should be chosen on the basis of the specific individual or population and should also recognize common comorbidities. For example, older adults aging in place are a common group receiving home modification services. Limitations they might experience include reduced strength and range of motion, poor visual acuity and contrast sensitivity, impaired gait and balance, and depression and impaired cognition. A baseline understanding of these factors is critical for therapists to make recommended changes. It is also important to understand, based on evidence, how these client factors may progress over time. In the case of older adults, it is possible that strength and mobility will not be static for a client who has severe arthritis. In some cases, a screening tool may indicate a need for a greater depth of assessment to support the development of an intervention plan. Occupational therapists working in specific areas of practice should develop a standard set of assessments they use to evaluate their clients' functional limitations.

Performance Patterns

Performance patterns include habits, routines, rituals, and roles (AOTA, 2014). Performance patterns can either support or hinder occupational performance.

The home environment is intimately connected with performance patterns. Many habits and routines acquire automaticity not only because they are performed repeatedly but also because they are repeated in a familiar and stable physical environment. Most ADLs and IADLs performed in the home form a complex tapestry of habits and routines occurring in consistent locations in the home and at consistent times of the day or week (Seamon, 2002). Many traditions are rituals involving not only consistent locations and times of day, week, month, or year but also people who consistently coparticipate in the rituals.

Habits

Habits are actions that are performed automatically, but to achieve automaticity, they must be performed repeatedly—that is, habitually. One challenge of assessment is that the habit itself may not become apparent until the specific cues (location, occasion, and tool) are present to prompt the habit. Discrepancies may be noted among self-reported abilities, habitual performance, and observed performance (Rogers et al., 2010).

Requesting demonstration of a task outside its habitual context—at an atypical location or even at an atypical time of day—may produce a performance that differs significantly from the habitual performance. Thus, performance elicited and demonstrated in an inpatient or an outpatient setting may not reflect the way the client has habitually performed the activity at home. In his studies of older adults, Rowles (1991) noted that activities performed habitually in the familiar environment may exceed the capabilities suggested by skills alone: "Repetition of actions within a familiar environment may allow a person to transcend sensory capabilities. . . . Such familiarity may be a factor in the strong attachment to home and reluctance to leave displayed by many elderly people" (pp. 267–268). Conversely, newly acquired skills or techniques newly learned in an unfamiliar environment are likely to be forgotten or supplanted by habitual ways of doing when the client returns to the home environment where the habit has been formed and refined for months, years, or even decades.

Habits may be dependent on individualized strategies and occur in specific locations or rooms in the home, so that the location, the strategies, and the actions making up the habit become integrated. If any aspect—strategy, location, or actions—is disrupted, the habit is disrupted. The performance and any outcome of the performance are also altered or disrupted. Often, it is not until a habit is disrupted that the habit itself becomes apparent.

Although change in a client's ability to execute actions of a habit will disrupt the habit, altering the tools or location, even to better match the client's abilities, will also disrupt the habit. Assessment of habit must consider the stability or flexibility of existing habits and how modification of the environment will affect them. Such assessment will also inform interventions related to training in use of the modifications, to reestablish habits integrating the modifications.

Routines

Routines are "established sequences of occupations or activities that provide a structure for daily life"

(AOTA, 2014, p. S8). Protraction or fragmentation of routines may occur when daily activities become difficult and activity demands exceed the effort available to execute them in a complete and timely sequence. When routines take too long, other activities may be disrupted. When routines require too much effort or energy, a client may be forced to perform the component activities in isolation, allowing time for rest before initiating the next activity. This strategy may be useful for conserving energy, but it may also disrupt other important daily life activities. Probing routines or disrupted routines identifies incompatibilities among activity and occupational demands, environment, and abilities. These incompatibilities may be resolved by home modifications that reduce the energy demands and sustain or reestablish a routine.

Roles

Roles are "sets of behaviors expected by society and shaped by culture and context; they may be further conceptualized and defined by a client" (AOTA, 2014, p. S8). Roles bridge the connection between what one does and who one is (Goffman, 1959). Each person inhabits multiple roles simultaneously. Some of the roles are familial: parent, child, sibling, grandparent, aunt, uncle, niece, and nephew. Other roles are related to civic and community relationships: neighbor, constituent, and voter. Some roles are related to relationships—friend, colleague, caregiver, and so forth—whereas others are related to interests and hobbies—collector, coach, quilter, bowler, or bridge player. Yet other roles are related to vocation: teacher, occupational therapist, engineer, attorney, or receptionist. Each role is associated with a constellation of activities.

Understanding a client's roles offers insight into the meaning and importance of specific activities. Roles not only correspond to a particular set of activities, they also suggest the meaning of the activities. For example, some clients consider preparing meals a routine daily activity, or IADL. However, for a client whose roles include cook, baker, or gourmet, activities such as preparing a homemade soup, kneading and baking bread, or preparing a family holiday dinner are not merely instrumental activities. For such a client, difficulty or risk associated with activities in the kitchen may threaten not only the ability to prepare meals but also an important aspect of how the client sees himself or herself.

Stark (2004) found that once activities are given up (because of an inability or risk associated with environmental barriers), a person is not likely to identify the activity as a problem. Probing activities in terms of roles may identify activities that the client wants to retain or resume that are central to a valued role.

Rituals

Rituals are "symbolic actions with spiritual, cultural, or social meaning. Rituals contribute to the client's identity and reinforcing values and beliefs" (Fiese, 2007; Segal, 2004; as cited in AOTA, 2014, p. S8). Rituals hold meanings common to participants—the achievement of graduation, the patriotism of an Independence Day parade, or the family bonds of a Thanksgiving meal. The constellation of activities and the shared cultural meanings both contribute to the ritual. Each participant may also associate the ritual with unique personal meanings in addition to the shared meanings.

Rituals may also be primarily personal—patterns of activity that hold particular meaning for the doer, those with whom the ritual is shared, or both. Many occupations that serve an instrumental purpose become rituals through the shared meaning-making of the occupation. For example, a parent reads to a toddler before bed to settle the child for sleep. Although the repeated performance of this activity may continue to serve the purpose of calming the child, the activity comes to hold special meaning for both the parent and the child, and the ritual is repeated, even when the child is already sleepy and needs no calming or the parent is tired or busy with other activities. The ritual persists when a second child comes along. It may persist as the once-read-to child assumes the role of parent and recalls the feelings associated with childhood bedtime reading. It may then persist across generations as the parent becomes a grandparent and makes meaning with the child's child by resuming or participating in the familiar ritual of the bedtime story (Siebert, 2008, p. 94).

Contexts and Environment

Occupational therapists acknowledge the influence of cultural, personal, temporal, and virtual contextual factors on occupations and activities. Environmental factors (physical and social) that support or hinder occupational performance should be identified throughout the evaluation and intervention process.

Physical

The physical spaces evaluated for home assessment can vary greatly. Homes evaluated during the home modification process can be single-family homes, stationary mobile homes, congregate living facilities including apartment complexes and college dormitories, recreational vehicles, and so forth. Community spaces adjacent to dwellings are also important aspects to evaluate for home modifications and can include the surrounding land such as the yard or garden; the structures within which the home is nested such as a lobby area or accessory buildings such as a garage or barn; or services used within a facility such as a laundry room, pool, or communal trash receptacle.

The United States has an incredible diversity of housing. A home modification may occur at a rural farm or a city apartment. Understanding where clients spend their time and conduct daily activities at home beyond the primary dwelling structure is an important aspect of the home modification process.

Physical environments also include transitional areas that link the home to the community. For example, routes to bus stops or driveways are important areas to evaluate. Aspects of these community areas such as safety and protection from weather are important considerations. It is important to understand where past, current, and desired occupations occur with the physical space and to evaluate each area during a home assessment. The assessment may thus involve evaluating multiple rooms (such as a bathroom) that have the same function.

The physical environment should also be evaluated for life safety issues. The ability to recognize and escape from dangerous situations should be an assessment priority. Each client should have a safety plan to address potential natural disasters specific to the region.

Cultural

The cultural context includes the customs, beliefs, activity patterns, behavior standards, and expectations accepted by the client and his or her cultural group. Some of these patterns of performance may be difficult when fit between a person and the home environment is decreased. For example, inaccessible entrances and bathrooms may make hosting or attending traditional family events difficult, if not impossible. Decorating for seasonal events may be impaired if a person is unable to reach high shelves or use a step stool safely. Cooking a meal for a family gathering becomes difficult when the kitchen appliances are not accessible for a person who uses a wheelchair for mobility. Simply greeting guests and visitors at the door can be challenging for someone with mobility limitations as a result of the floor covering or fine motor limitations that hinder operation of the door handle.

Occupational therapy practitioners provide culturally responsive care by displaying an awareness of and sensitivity to the client's cultural beliefs about health and how culture may influence the client's typical activity patterns and occupations. For example, if the client and family members believe that the family is the primary care provider, they may not value modifications to the home that would promote independence. By engaging in culturally competent care, occupational therapists will incorporate the person's values, beliefs, ways of life, and practices into a mutually acceptable intervention plan.

Personal

Personal attributes, such as gender, socioeconomic status, age, clinical course of a health condition, and level of education, all factor into the evaluation of the home environment and subsequent intervention process. For instance, the stage and prognosis of a health condition will determine whether home modifications may be temporary, permanent, or phased in over time as a condition progresses. Likewise, a client's occupational profile may be influenced by age, gender, level of education, and other personal factors, and the fit between the client and the environment will therefore be unique in each case.

Socioeconomic status can also affect a home assessment and intervention plan. For example, most third-party payers do not reimburse commonly recommended home modifications such as adding a ramp to an entryway or installing grab bars in a shower area; thus, these modifications would be out-of-pocket expenses. It is important for occupational therapy practitioners to understand the potential financial barriers associated with home modifications and either offer alternative strategies that would achieve the same objective or advocate for the client to obtain the necessary services or devices.

Aesthetic preferences are another personal consideration that occupational therapy practitioners should take into account during home assessment and intervention planning. A client may have a strong affinity for particular pieces of furniture, a particular room arrangement, or even a certain wall color. Again, these types of personal preferences will influence occupational therapy practitioners' clinical decision making and intervention planning.

Temporal

On a large scale, *temporal context* may refer to the time in a person's life at which the condition necessitating a home evaluation occurred, such as adulthood or late adulthood. It can also refer to the stage of progression of the health condition, which influences clinical decision making about options for home modification or other intervention strategies. For example, a client in the early stages of cognitive decline may have more intervention options than a client in the later stages.

The time of the year and time of the day are relevant when conducting a home evaluation, and occupational therapy practitioners may consider this influence of time as part of the temporal context of engagement in occupation. When occupational therapists conduct a home evaluation in a northern climate that has distinct changes of season, they must take into account how each season may influence the environment and make appropriate recommendations for snow, rain, heat, and other weather conditions. Likewise, the time of the day at which a client typically performs desired occupations should be considered so that appropriate lighting recommendations can be made.

Social

The social environment or context includes a client's social network of friends, family, groups, and organizations with whom the client has contact. These social relationships carry expectations for interaction, and people with decreased safety and independence in performing occupations of choice in their home environment may experience hindrances in the social environment. For instance, difficulty answering the front door, accessing the telephone, or navigating an entryway to get out of the house can all contribute to social isolation. Clients who have physical difficulty getting in and out of the house may drift away from family and friends, and they may struggle to remain in their social roles (e.g., card groups or church activities may

be discontinued because of their inability to attend regularly scheduled events out of the home).

Other family members living in the home environment or those who come into the home to provide care are also a part of the social context. The degree to which these individuals are in agreement with the proposed intervention will also influence home assessment and intervention planning. Simply stated, their preferences for modifications may be different from the client's preferences. Although a tub transfer bench may be one strategy that addresses safety and independence in showering, other family members may perceive it as interfering with their own showering activities. Similarly, a family member may not want kitchen items rearranged to promote access from a seated position because he or she routinely prepares most of the meals from a standing position. Occupational therapy practitioners need to be mindful of how even a simple home modification recommendation may create a significant incompatibility with another family member's habits or roles.

Virtual

The virtual environment is one in which communication occurs in the absence of physical contact or proximity. In the area of home modifications, occupational therapists may need to evaluate the occupant's use of electronic devices and other technology to interact in the virtual environment (e.g., use of a personal computer, landline or mobile phone, tablet, television). It is important to determine both what types of devices the client is using in the home setting and where in the home these devices are used. The goal for assessment of the virtual context is to ensure that the intervention plan for modifying the home supports the use of the electronic devices that promote socialization by means of virtual communication. For example, for a person who regularly uses a desktop computer to participate in an online community, the occupational therapist would evaluate the client's mobility, seating options, and access options.

Considerations in Assessments

Ownership and Control

A key question must be answered during the evaluation process: Who owns or controls the dwelling unit? The answer will have an important bearing on any proposed modifications. If the client owns the dwelling, then the client can give the final authorization for most modifications. However, if the client is a renter or lives in cooperative housing, the owner or ownership association has the final decision regarding any modifications that alter the structure or fixtures of the home.

Other entities may have authority over implementation of modifications. Changes to the structure, fixtures, or utilities may require authorization or permitting from local authorities. Changes to the home's appearance may require the authorization of a homeowners' association or historic commission.

Payment and Reimbursement

Although detailed funding and reimbursement strategies are beyond the scope of this practice guideline, most equipment, fixtures, or structural changes are not covered by traditional third-party payers, such as Medicare or private health insurance. However, sources of funding may be available on the basis of a client's age, health condition, location, or income. Examples of such funding include Medicaid waiver programs, home and community block grant programs, charitable or civic organizations serving people with specific health conditions, and housing rehabilitation and repair organizations.

Occupational therapy evaluation and intervention to identify, implement, and train a client in use of home modifications is typically covered by Medicare and other insurers if other coverage criteria are met (usually the presence of an associated health condition and a physician referral or order). It is always best to check the specific exclusions of a particular insurance. When no health insurance or other funding is available, a client may opt to pay out of pocket for home modification evaluation, implementation, or training. It is important to note that fabrication or installation of home modifications is not within the scope of reimbursable occupational therapy services and must be paid for by the client or another party, such as a local service organization or a special government program. A description of services by *CPT* code is provided in Appendix B.

Consultation vs. Direct Service

Sometimes organizations involved in providing home modifications may seek an occupational therapist to consult with the organization. In these circumstances, the person receiving the home modifications is the organization's client, and the organization is the occupational therapist's client. In these circumstances, the organization may seek an occupational therapist to evaluate, assist in planning modifications, or train the client to use the modifications.

Rebuilding Together is an example of an organization that works with occupational therapists in this capacity. Similar arrangements may be sought by liability insurance case managers or attorneys involved in liability litigation on behalf of the person needing home modifications.

Home Modifications, Home Audits, and Accessibility

Home modifications practice is sometimes confused with home audit or with accessibility consulting. Although home audit and accessibility also pertain to the environment, home modifications practice differs significantly from either of these activities.

Home modifications vs. safety or accessibility audits

A wide variety of checklists and similar tools are available to identify safety concerns or to determine whether a wheeled mobility user can maneuver in a space or access a feature. Often, these audits can be conducted without a specific client present. Such audits do not take into consideration the unique abilities, preferences, habits, or needs of a specific person but are instead based on generalities or general rules.

In contrast, occupational therapy home modifications practice begins with the client and the client's specific activities in the home, identifying the specific incompatibilities affecting the client's engagement and modifications that fit the needs and preferences of the client and other occupants of the home. Home modifications practice also includes training the client or caregiver as necessary to ensure that modifications, once implemented, are effective and integrated.

Access and housing laws

Federal laws are often cited in reference to home modifications. The two most commonly cited are the Americans With Disabilities Act of 1990 (ADA) as amended and the Fair Housing Act Amendments of 1988 (FHAA). The ADA is a civil rights law that applies to many aspects of the built environment but does not apply to most private dwellings. However, private dwellings are subject to local and state building codes.

The FHAA are relevant to home modifications for clients who are renters in the private rental market. Landlords cannot prohibit renters from making reasonable modifications to the rental unit to accommodate a disability, and this law does not require landlords or owners to pay for such accommodations. However, it does permit the landlord to require the tenant to restore the rental unit to its original (unmodified) condition or to charge the tenant for the cost of restoring the rental unit to its original state (e.g., remove the accommodation) on vacating the unit. The landlord also has the option of retaining the accommodation and not charging for restoration to the move-in condition. If a person lives in owner-occupied rental housing of four or fewer units or a single-family dwelling and the owner possesses no more than three such units (wherever located), the FHAA do not apply.

Impact of poor housing

Poor housing conditions influence function, health, and safety and should be considered during occupational therapy home modifications. Hazards linked with poor housing are associated with a range of negative health consequences and safety threats (Krieger & Higgins, 2002). These hazards include, but are not limited to, dampness, mold, temperature extremes, noise, insecurity, overcrowding, and fire safety. Costs associated with poor housing are poor health, social isolation, increased medical expense, and more frequent accidents (Nicol et al., 2010). If poor housing conditions are present, the hazards may need to be addressed before the intervention or included in it.

Occupational therapy practitioners may need to work with an interprofessional team or report unsafe conditions to appropriate entities to resolve poor housing conditions. In some states, occupational therapy practitioners are mandated reporters of hazardous situations that pose a danger to self or others (e.g., a person who has severe dementia living alone in poor housing) and are required to report unsafe conditions to local authorities.

Intervention

Types of Interventions

Occupational therapy practitioners also consider the type of intervention when determining the most effective intervention plan for a given client in need of home modifications. Therapeutic use of self is an integral part of the occupational therapy process, "which allows occupational therapy practitioners to develop and manage their therapeutic relationship with clients by using narrative and clinical reasoning; empathy; and a client-centered, collaborative approach to service delivery." (Taylor & Van Puymbroeck, 2013, as cited in AOTA, 2014, p. S12).

Intervention Approaches

Once occupational therapists have identified targeted goals in collaboration with the client or family, he or she determines the intervention approach that is best suited to address the goals. Some approaches may be more appropriate at some times than at others. The intervention approaches most commonly used by occupational therapy practitioners providing home modifications are as follows:

- *Prevent,* an intervention approach designed to address clients with or without disability who are at risk for occupational performance problems (Dunn McClain, Brown, & Youngstrom, 1998); for example, intervention to prevent falls, prevent functional decline, or prevent caregiver stress or burnout. Providing a home hazard assessment and barrier removal for older adults at risk for a fall (Gillespie et al., 2012) has demonstrated a reduction in community-based falls.
- *Modify* activity demands and the contexts in which activities are performed to support safe, independent performance of valued activities within the constraints of motor, cognitive, or perceptual limitations; for example, modifying the home environment by reducing environmental barriers such as stairs without railings or lack of grab bars in the shower.
- *Create* or *promote* a healthy and satisfying lifestyle that includes adherence to medication routine, appropriate diet, appropriate levels of physical activity, and satisfying levels of engagement in social relationships and activities by providing enriched contextual and activity experiences that will enhance performance for all persons in the natural contexts of life (Dunn et al.,1998).
- *Maintain* performance and health by providing environmental support to facilitate performance of daily activities, increase safety (e.g., reduce falls), and reduce caregiver burden.

Home modification can include changes to the physical environment (both the layout of the space and the products and controls in the environment), the addition of adaptive equipment to compensate for functional loss, and the addition of personal support that may be needed to achieve occupational performance goals. Often, a blend of all three approaches is used in successful intervention. Table 4 illustrates examples of these various approaches, used singly or in combination, to address selected occupational performance problems.

Adaptive equipment
Adaptive equipment is freestanding, meaning it is not part of the structure of the dwelling (Mann,

Table 4. Selected Home Modification Solutions, by Occupational Performance Issue

Problem	Architectural Solution	Adapted Equipment	Behavioral Change Solution
Client unable to transfer to or from bathtub	Replace tub with no-step shower, or install a ceiling-mounted lift.	Install grab bars and transfer bench.	Use caregiver assistance to transfer or sponge bathe at sink.
Doorway not wide enough for wheelchair passage	Widen doorway or add alternate doorway opening.	Install swing-clear hinges.	Reconfigure spaces in the home so room is no longer essential.
Client unable to access items in kitchen cupboards	Install pantry or other storage at accessible height, or install pull-out shelves (in base cupboards).	Use reacher to retrieve items.	Rearrange so items used most often are within reach on accessible shelves or counters.
Client unable to transfer to or from standard toilet	Install 18-inch-high toilet and grab bars or toilet arms.	Install toilet elevator or riser, or use bedside commode over toilet.	Use caregiver assistance for transfer.
Client unable to independently navigate stairs	Install hand rail on both sides of stairs, or install additional lighting along stairs.	Install stair glide system.	Relocate bedroom to accessible level of home.

Hurren, Tomita, Bengali, & Steinfeld, 1994). Examples include a bathtub transfer bench and a handheld shower for someone who is unable to stand while showering. Adaptive equipment can include specialized durable medical equipment such as a toilet safety frame, specially designed devices such as a long-handled reacher or pick-up tool, or commercially marketed products that support performance such as a robotic vacuum cleaner (Kraskowsky & Finlayson, 2001).

Architectural modifications

Architectural modifications refer to additions, deletions, or reconfigurations of the structure. These modifications range from simple modifications, such as adding grab bars or rails at an entryway, to complex modifications, such as replacing a tub with a walk-in shower or the major remodeling of a kitchen to make it accessible for a wheeled mobility user.

Behavioral strategies

Behavioral strategies involve modifying the way the person interacts with the environment. Occupational therapists also modify how people use the physical environment by providing education and training to change how the client interacts with the environment to ensure safety in the home. Occupational therapists may teach a client to use existing environmental features in ways that make it safer or easier to perform daily activities. For example, occupational therapists may identify illuminating a stairway before ascending or descending as a strategy to reduce risk of injury.

Application of strategies

The environment can also be changed in multiple ways to reduce barriers in each of these strategy categories. Occupational therapists can add features to an environment (additional handrails), remove features from an environment (remove a threshold from a doorway), or modify existing features (reduce the tension on a door opener). Features of the environment that are barriers to one person may serve as supports to another. The goal of the intervention process is to achieve optimal compatibility between the client's abilities and the environment. In circumstances in which multiple occupants of the home will have to interact with the modified features, the intervention must be compatible with the abilities of all users.

Use of a Team Approach

One of occupational therapists' most important roles is educating clients about how to solve barriers and what is feasible in their unique situation. An intervention plan for home modifications should be developed with the entire home modification team. The first step involves identifying potential solutions that enable the client to meet occupational goals and are feasible given the unique personal and environmental factors relevant to the situation. The intervention plan will include potential modification strategies that would address the occupational performance issues identified, and relevant members of the intervention team should discuss the expected outcome of the intervention. Agreement on the final intervention plan should be documented and an interprofessional plan to implement the strategies developed.

In a referral arrangement, occupational therapy practitioners must obtain the client's permission to share client information with other professionals whose services are engaged to implement the plan. Occupational therapy practitioners are also obligated to disclose to the client any financial relationship that exists between the practitioner and other professionals or organizations to whom the referral is made (AOTA, 2010).

Intervention Plan

As a part of the occupational therapy process, occupational therapists develop an intervention plan that considers the client's goals, values, and beliefs; the client's health and well-being; the client's performance skills and performance patterns; collective influence of the context, environment,

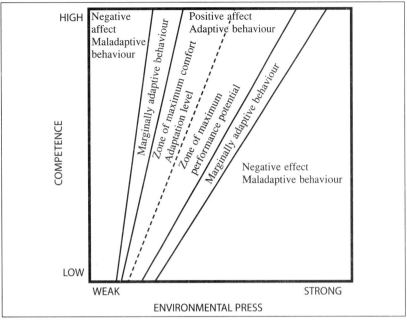

Figure 3. Environmental Press

Source. Adapted with permission from Lawton, M. P., & Nahemow, L. (1973). Ecology and the aging process. In C. Eisdorfer & M. P. Lawton (Eds.), *The psychology of adult development and aging* (pp. 619–674). Washington, DC: American Psychological Association.

and client factors on the client's performance; the activity demands; and the context of service delivery in which the intervention is provided (e.g., caregiver expectations, organization's purpose, payer's requirements, or applicable regulations; AOTA, 2014). The intervention plan outlines and guides the therapist's actions and is based on the best available evidence to meet the identified outcomes. There are often multiple ways to reduce or eliminate environmental barriers. The intervention planning process involves understanding the client's unique circumstances to present a set of strategies that are appropriate for the client's situation.

Foundations for Intervention Planning

In delivering home modification interventions, occupational therapists rely on a set of foundation skills to effectively develop an evidence-based intervention plan. These foundations include application of theoretical approaches, context-based task analysis, activity demands, and the use of a client-centered approach to intervention.

Theoretical Approaches

Most efficacious home modification interventions are based on a competence–press framework (Lawton & Nahemow, 1973). *Environmental press* (Lawton & Nahemow, 1973) is a term often used by professionals to communicate the effect of activity demands associated with the physical environment. Lawton and Nahemow's (1973) ecological model conceptualized the person–physical environment relationship as an interaction between a person's competencies (similar to client factors and performance skills) and the demands of the physical environment, or environmental press. Figure 3 illustrates this relationship.

Applying Lawton and Nahemow's (1973) theory, if a misfit exists between a client's capacity and his or her environment because the press is too great, occupational therapists reduce the demands of the environment to match the client's abilities. For example, if a client has limited mobility and cannot step into a bathtub, an occupational therapist may add a tub transfer bench to reduce the environment's press or demand to match the person's capacity. Similarly, if a misfit occurs because the press is not strong enough (e.g., resulting in boredom), home modifications can be used to add complexity to the environment using physical or cognitive challenges or opportunities for interaction. For example, if an older adult is lonely or bored at home, adding complexity by increasing leisure activity choices may increase the environment's complexity and result in a better fit between capacity and press.

The use of home modifications is a compensatory strategy. Although it is possible to create challenge in the environment to increase a client's capacity (Clemson et al., 2012), home modifications are in most cases designed to reduce environmental press.

Task Analysis

Task analysis for occupational therapy is the process of analyzing the dynamic relationship between people and their occupations within environments or performance contexts (Watson & Llorens, 1997), which differs from activity analysis in that it is performed in context rather than out of context. The analysis generally involves identifying and describing the occupation and the demands of the task and evaluating the relevant contextual issues. Occupational therapists compare the typical demands of the occupation with the client's unique abilities and then examine the environment for existing barriers and supports. The conceptual framework for developing home modification, developed by Connell and Sanford (1997), is useful for task analysis. It provides an organizing scheme to systematically analyze environmental features into relevant spaces, products, and controls.

Occupational therapists can conduct task analysis at each of these organizational levels of the environment (spaces, products, controls) and address barriers present at each level. For example, the layout of a bathroom (space) may be modified to increase the space available for a wheelchair turning radius, the toilet (product) may be modified to increase its height, or the type of toilet flusher

(control) may be modified to facilitate limited fine motor function.

Activity Demands

Determining whether a client may be able to complete an activity depends not only on the client's performance skills, performance patterns, and client factors but also on the demands the activity itself places on him or her. *Activity demands* are aspects of the activity that include the tools and resources needed to carry out the activity; the physical space and social demands required by the activity; sequence and timing of the steps or the necessary procedures and rules of the activity; and the required actions and performance skills needed to engage in the given activity.

Activity demands are assessed primarily through the process of activity analysis, which has no formal assessment tools associated with it. The following paragraphs address the various types of activity demands and provide strategies and examples of assessment for each type.

Space demands
Space demands are the spatial requirements of an activity—the arrangement of the space and its properties, including illumination, ventilation, and ambient sound. Two common reasons why spatial requirements increase are (1) use of an assistive mobility device (e.g., walker, rollator, wheelchair) or a transfer assist device (e.g., floor-based lift) and (2) the need for human assistance or caregiving during an activity. When assessing the space required for the activity, occupational therapists must consider the additional space occupied by the device, the assistant, or both, as well as the space required to approach or access the activity area and the space required during engagement in the activity. For example, a bathroom may offer adequate space for a client using a walker to access the fixtures and maneuver between them, but if the doorway to the bathroom is too narrow for the client to enter the bathroom while using the walker,

then all activities performed in the bathroom will be affected because the space demands exceed the space available in the existing environment.

Illumination, temperature, ambient sound, and humidity are less obvious properties of an activity space that may affect the client's performance. For example, a client may report having problems managing medication, specifically in discriminating one medication vial from another. When directly assessed during the day, the client may have no difficulty performing the task. However, more specific probing may reveal that the problem arises when the client takes medication in the evening. This additional information indicates that illumination may be a factor, confirmed by presence of a single lamp with a 60-watt bulb. Inadequate task lighting would thus be identified as an activity demand contributing to the client's difficulty.

Social demands
The social demands of an activity take on special significance when assessing activities conducted at home. Introducing objects to the home that the client associates with other contexts or that have meanings incompatible with the client's sense of home may result in the client rejecting those objects. For example, a client may have no objection to using assistive devices or durable medical equipment in an inpatient or outpatient setting but may express discomfort or resistance to using or even having the same device in the home.

The client's social and cultural contexts inform the social demands of the activity. The social context encompasses societal conventions as well as the preferences, needs, and expectations of those living in the home. A more subtle aspect of social demands to consider in the home is the impact of modifying activity demands on others who reside in the home. For example, in the inpatient setting, it is common to recommend or even order a raised toilet seat or a three-in-one bedside commode for a client to use on discharge to home to reduce the motor activity demands associated with toilet transfers. If the client shares the bathroom with other occupants, however, the presence of the device may be inconvenient or undesirable. This circumstance may lead to one of two undesirable situations: (1) the client accepting the device but other occupants developing ill feelings toward the client because of the inconvenience or (2) the client refusing the device in anticipation of such a response from the other occupants.

Required actions and performance skills
This aspect of activity demands includes the motor, process, and social interaction aspects of a given activity. Assessment involves analysis of the specific activities that the client identifies as problematic. Often the client is able to identify the specific required actions or performance skills that are contributing to the problem, such as having to bend or reach to perform selected aspects of an activity or having to discriminate visual information that exceeds the client's visual acuity. At other times, the client may identify an activity as a problem but be unable to identify why it is a problem. In many cases, the unidentified demand is related to the activity's sequencing, timing, or energy demands, for example, a client expresses frustration with being unable to perform a simple activity such as making a cold lunch but does not appreciate the energy demands associated with being on his or her feet in the kitchen for the 10 minutes required to complete the tasks.

Tools and resources needed to perform the activity
Tools, materials, and equipment used during an activity contribute to activity demands. The tools for the activity must be available and accessible. Their inherent properties (e.g., weight, texture, appearance, sound) contribute to activity demands by requiring various responses, or inhibition of responses, from the client. For example, a cast iron skillet may be a client's preferred tool for cooking eggs. The weight and the heat-conducting proper-

ties of a cast iron skillet impose specific demands on the client's sensory, motor, and cognitive abilities to avoid dropping it or burning a hand when handling the heated skillet. During task analysis, tools can be conceived in terms of the level of environmental press they offer.

Occupational performance occurs at the intersection of a person's competencies and the magnitude of the environmental press (Iwarsson & Stähl, 2003). When environmental press is strong and personal competencies are relatively low, occupational performance is affected negatively. In this circumstance, when activities in the home become difficult, unsafe, or impossible, the need for home modifications often becomes apparent. The concept of environmental press is used by a variety of professionals who may be part of the interprofessional home modifications team. To enhance team communication, occupational therapists working in home modifications should be familiar with environmental press and be at ease communicating findings in terms of either activity demands or environmental press.

Client-Centered Approach

Finally, in determining intervention strategies, it is imperative that occupational therapists act in a client-centered manner or risk the client's abandoning expensive intervention strategies. In most cases, multiple solutions exist for each identified environmental barrier. For example, the occupational performance issue of obtaining a meal for a person who has limited use of the left upper extremity can be solved by kitchen modification, use of adaptive equipment and task modification, or provision of a meal delivery service.

The type of intervention must be based on the person's preferences. If the person wants to cook for himself or herself alone in the home, a kitchen modification may be necessary, whereas if the person lives with a caregiver, he or she may be satisfied with adaptive equipment and set up at the kitchen table. Presenting clients with a range of

options allows them to weigh the costs in relation to their needs, priorities, aesthetic tastes, family goals, and values. Occupational therapists' role is to present clients with information about potential interventions and their expected outcomes to assist them in their decision about modifications of their home environment.

Considerations During Intervention Planning

The decisions occupational therapists make regarding which type of modification to recommend are dependent on multiple factors. The results of the comprehensive assessment (of the person, the environment, and occupational performance), the client's occupational performance goals, and the personal and environmental factors that influence the client's life will have an impact on home modification intervention. Attention to these considerations is essential for delivery of an effective client-centered intervention that has high adherence (Stark et al., 2013).

Type and Ownership of Home

The type and ownership of a home are important considerations. The considerable structural and organizational characteristics of individual homes present a set of benefits and challenges that must be a primary consideration in intervention. Home types may include single detached homes, mobile homes, houseboats, attached homes, apartments, and condominiums. Homes can be designed for single or multiple families, can include retrofitted loft spaces in large cities, or can be large single-family homes in rural farming communities. Most homes were designed without features that support the performance of adults with newly acquired disabilities or older adults aging in place who would benefit from such modifications (Tabbarah et al., 2000). Although no policy mandates modifications in either privately owned or rental housing, local jurisdictions may provide tax incentives for accessible features in homes.

Antidiscrimination statutes that apply to multifamily rental housing are not applicable to some single-family or small multifamily units. In some cases, only limited interventions are possible because of legal or policy regulations for both private and rented homes. Thus, a landlord may legally prohibit the addition of a ramp to a single, freestanding small rental unit. Practitioners should be aware of local, state, and national statutes and be prepared to recommend that their clients seek more information.

Condition and Layout

The condition and layout of the home may influence the type of modifications that are possible. For example, older homes with deteriorating infrastructure may not support home modification interventions. The layout and space available may influence the possible solutions that can be used. Small spaces may prohibit the installation of ramps, which require more square footage than stairs or lifts. For complex home modifications, occupational therapists should work with the interprofessional team to understand building code requirements and infrastructure issues that influence decisions about the possible interventions.

Needs of All Residents

Occupational therapists must also consider other residents or occupants in the home who may be influenced by or who will influence environmental modifications. Clients often have family members who live with them or visit on a frequent basis, and clients living in multifamily housing units may share common space with other residents. The needs of small children, pets, and caregivers must be considered in intervention planning.

Cost and Client Preferences

Home modifications can be costly. The resources available to install the home modification (covered by insurance, paid out of pocket, or provided through a social services agency) should be a consideration when developing an intervention plan. It is important to offer estimates of costs when discussing intervention options so clients can make informed choices about which interventions to select.

Because renovations can be costly and permanent, it is important to plan for modifications that will continue to meet the needs of the client (and the client's family members) over time. Future marketability of the home may be an important consideration for the client. Universally designed modifications may appeal to a broader audience and make the home more marketable.

Occupational therapists should consider the possible course of a chronic disease or how a person with a disability might age and recommend modifications accordingly. Interventions should target the client's current and future abilities so they do not become obsolete, and occupational therapists may educate clients about the modifications' long-term feasibility. In some cases, clients may decide to move to a more compatible home in the community rather than invest resources in home modifications.

Home is often considered a reflection of self (Cooper Marcus, 1997; Dovey, 1985). Some clients will refuse to implement home modifications because of the image the modifications project. In some cases (e.g., a ramp to a front door), clients may worry that modifications advertise disability or vulnerability. In other cases, appearance of equipment or changes perceived as medical may not be aesthetically acceptable to clients or their family. Understanding a client's preferences for the appearance of the home modifications is important.

The requirements of the modification with regard to upkeep, use, and maintenance are a consideration that must be balanced with the client's abilities and willingness. Clients who are averse to technology may require a simplified strategy. Technology that requires an energy source or maintenance may be too difficult for the client to manage independently. In addition, literacy levels and understanding how to manage and operate adaptive equipment or a complicated modification may be a consideration.

In some cases, clients may prefer to rely on the personal assistance of their family members. In other cases, they may prefer complete independence in tasks. Establishing an acceptable level of personal assistance for the client and the resources to provide that support (either paid or unpaid) will influence the intervention plan.

What financial resources are available to carry out the intervention plan should be established. Most home modification interventions are paid for by the client or homeowner. Determining the personal resources the client is willing to commit to a home modification as well as the community and social resources available will support the development of a realistic intervention plan. The occupational therapist's role should be to describe the potential home modifications that are possible and allow the client to identify the resources for obtaining the intervention. Occupational therapists should not make assumptions regarding a client's ability to pay but should identify community resources that may offer additional financial support.

Culture

In some cases, cultural values and norms may influence the acceptability of home modifications. For example, in some cultures, offering assistance to an older member of the family is a way of honoring that person. The intervention plan should reflect these values. Modified assistance, safety, and caregiver self-efficacy may be the target goals instead of independence in performing the activity.

Intervention Implementation

The intervention will vary greatly depending on the setting and the role of the clinician. Typical interventions involve an evaluation encounter, one or more encounters to consult with the intervention team, an encounter to review potential options for interventions and finalize the intervention plan, and then encounters as appropriate to teach the client to use the interventions effectively and to evaluate outcomes.

Once an intervention plan has been established and approved by the client (and, if appropriate, family and caregivers) and other team members, intervention implementation can commence. Occupational therapists will communicate and collaborate with the team to understand the timeline for installation of the home modifications. Occupational therapists' role in carrying out the intervention can involve facilitating the procurement of adapted equipment or medical equipment, monitoring the construction of architectural modifications to ensure that the intervention plan is implemented as planned, and training the client to use the new modifications safely and effectively. It may be necessary to modify the intervention plan as the intervention progresses as a result of unexpected findings during construction. Changes in the client's abilities or failure of the intervention to fully address the client's need may also result in revisions to the intervention plan.

Once the modifications are in place, the focus of intervention is on establishing or reestablishing performance of the occupations with the new environmental supports in place to develop new habits and routines. This phase of intervention will vary depending on the complexity of the interventions and the length of time needed to install them. Training in the use of the home modifications is provided to achieve both effective and habitual or integrated performance. To achieve effective performance, the practitioner instructs the client (and caregiver) in how to use the intervention to achieve occupational performance goals. The occupational therapy practitioner may demonstrate how to use the intervention and provide an opportunity for the client to use the modification while the practitioner is present. In this way, the practitioner verifies that the client's understanding of the instruction and performance are adequate for him or her to use the home modifications safely and effectively.

To achieve habitual or integrated performance, occupational therapists evaluate the client's use of the modifications in light of existing routines and habits. In nearly all cases, home modifications require some change in existing habits or routines. Table 4 provides examples of common functional performance problems and home modification strategies to resolve those problems. Table 4 also illustrates the role of training in relation to habits and routines.

The behavioral change solutions in Table 4 clearly involve altering a client's existing habits and routines. If a caregiver is involved, implementing behavior change solutions also alters that person's existing habits or routines. Some modifications reduce risk or dependence but involve an entirely new way of performing an activity. Adaptive equipment or architectural changes also involve new ways of doing that disrupt existing habits and routines. In some cases, a modification involves an entirely new way of performing an activity.

Training may address learning to use the modification but, more important, training addresses the revision of an established habit or routine. For example, a client who receives a tub transfer bench may demonstrate the ability to use the device when a demonstration is requested. However, because it is likely that the client has habitually stepped over the side of the tub for years (or did so for years before the task became too difficult or risky), successful integration involves revising the habit of approaching the tub and spontaneously attempting to step over the side of it and establishing the habit of approaching the tub and then turning around to sit on the transfer bench.

Even when the client or caregiver demonstrates the ability to use the modification, such use will initially require conscious attention to the new way of doing. With repetition, the use of the modification becomes more habitual, and the activity requires little or no conscious attention and, often, less time to complete. In such cases, intervention may include both training in the use of the modifications and additional follow-up contacts to verify that use of the modifications has become routine. If the client is experiencing difficulty routinizing the use of the modifications, occupational therapists may provide additional instruction, demonstration, or adaptation to achieve routinization.

If modifications apply to multiple occupations, integrating the modifications may require not only learning to use the modifications and making their use habitual but also reestablishing entire routines. For example, if bathroom modifications have been made to enable the client to perform personal care without assistance, a new unassisted personal care routine may emerge that differs significantly from the previous assisted routine. Fully routinizing the use of extensive modifications may require a period of adjustment as the client masters the use of the devices, the use becomes habitual, and the sequence of affected activities comes together as a seamless routine.

Intervention Review

Intervention review is a continuous process of reevaluating and reviewing the intervention plan, the effectiveness of its delivery, progress toward targeted outcomes, and the need for future occupational therapy and referrals to other agencies or professionals (AOTA, 2014). Reevaluation may involve readministering assessments used at the time of initial evaluation, a satisfaction questionnaire completed by the client, or questions that evaluate each goal (Minkel, 1996). Reevaluation normally substantiates progress toward goal attainment, indicates any change in functional status, and directs modification of the intervention plan, if necessary (Moyers & Dale, 2007).

During the occupational therapy process for home modification, intervention review occurs as the home modifications are being installed and the client is learning how to integrate the changes in the environment into his or her daily routine. The goals that were established as part of the intervention plan should periodically be reviewed to ensure that the plan and its implementation are aligned with the goals as implementation proceeds.

For example, a client with mobility limitations resulting from hip arthroplasty had a desired goal of completing the task of toileting independently; however, the 14-inch height of the existing toilet limited independence in this task. The chosen intervention was to install an elevated toilet seat with attached arms to achieve a 19-inch toilet height and assist in the transition on and off the toilet. After the modification was installed and the occupational therapist provided training in the use of the seat, the intervention was reviewed. The occupational therapist may directly assess the client performing the transfer or the toileting task to determine whether the desired outcome has been achieved or elicit the client's perspective to determine whether the intervention is satisfactory and meets the client's desired goal. If the client is not able to complete toileting successfully with the modification or finds the modifications objectionable, the intervention plan may be revised to include a different modification strategy (e.g., comfort-height toilet and grab bar installation) to achieve the desired result.

When the selected intervention strategies include major home renovation, the intervention review is also an opportunity for occupational therapists to meet with the home modification team to determine whether the renovation is progressing according to plan. Unanticipated events and circumstances such as unforeseen structural issues once walls are removed can necessitate changes to construction or renovation projects. The intervention review provides an opportunity to ensure that the efforts of all team members are directed toward target outcomes, even when intervention strategies must be modified to account for unforeseen obstacles.

Targeting of Outcomes

A focus on outcomes is interwoven throughout the process of occupational therapy (AOTA, 2014). Occupational therapists should contribute their client data and perspective to comprehensive team-based outcome assessments. Occupational therapists and occupational therapy assistants document outcomes in discharge evaluations or discontinuation notes (AOTA, 2013b). This documentation should be completed "within the time frames, formats, and standards established by practice settings, agencies, external accreditation programs, and payers" (AOTA, 2010, p. S109).

Targeting outcomes is a process that begins at the time of the initial evaluation when occupational therapists collaborate with the client to identify the goals of the occupational therapy process. It includes these steps:

1. Selecting types of outcomes and measures, including but not limited to occupational performance, health and wellness, participation, prevention, role competence, and quality of life; and
2. Using outcomes to measure progress and adjust goals and interventions (AOTA, 2014).

Goals may be revised during the occupational therapy home modification process as the client's goals, context, and abilities change.

Several types of occupational therapy outcomes can be measured as they pertain to the home modification process. Areas of outcome measurement within occupational therapy include occupational performance, prevention, health and wellness, quality of life, participation, role competence, well-being, and occupational justice (AOTA, 2014). The selection of the appropriate outcome monitoring tools will depend on the type of outcomes being tracked.

Occupational Performance

The installation of home modifications is not the end goal of the occupational therapy process;

rather, it is the ability to use the modification to support engagement in the occupations of daily life. Several formal assessment tools are available to assist in the measurement of occupational performance, including the COPM (Law et al., 2005), the I–HOPE (Stark et al., 2010), and the Activity Card Sort (Baum & Edwards, 2008). Both the COPM and the I–HOPE allow clients to rate their own performance and their satisfaction with performance of priority occupations before and after implementation of interventions (Law et al., 2005; Stark et al., 2010).

The Activity Card Sort allows clients to identify current engagement in occupations and, when used as an outcome measure, would thus indicate which occupations a client is able to participate in that he or she was not able to before the implementation of intervention strategies (Baum & Edwards, 2008). Alternatively, occupational therapists can use informal observation as a means of measuring occupational performance; however, it should be noted that this type of outcome monitoring is more difficult to aggregate to collect meaningful information about the effectiveness of a home modification program and to inform evidence-based practice.

Prevention

Home modification interventions may also contribute to the prevention of injury, disease, or further disability; therefore, measurement at the prevention level may also be desirable. For example, replacing carpet with vinyl or hardwood flooring may prevent unnecessary falls for a client who uses a walker to assist with mobility. Similarly, the installation of grab bars in the toilet and tub areas of the bathroom improves safety and prevents accidents. Measurement at the prevention level is not only valuable in documenting the effectiveness of occupational therapy intervention for an individual client, but it also aids in communicating the value of occupational therapy services to society in terms of reduced institutionalization and health care cost savings.

Health and Wellness

The outcome of the home modifications may also be measured by determining the impact that the modification has on the health and wellness of the client, caregiver, or both. For example, strong evidence exists that home modification interventions reduce the number of falls that occur in the home setting and improve the ability to provide care to others in the home (see Table 5 for a list of recommendations for evidence-based occupational therapy interventions). These outcomes positively affect the physical, mental, and emotional health and well-being of both the client and the care provider and may reduce potential clinic, hospital, or emergency room visits. Self-report tools may be used to track the number of falls in the home for a predefined period of time both before and after a home modification intervention; likewise, self-report tools may be used to assess the effect that a home modification has on the care provider.

Quality of Life

Quality of life can be defined as a client's dynamic appraisal of life satisfaction (perception of progress toward identified goals), self-concept (the composite of beliefs and feelings about himself or herself), health and functioning (including health status, self-care capabilities), and socioeconomic factors (e.g., vocation, education, income; adapted from Radomski, 1995). Home modifications may dramatically affect a client's sense of hope if they enable the client to remain in his or her own home rather than transition to institutionalized care. They can provide a sense of life satisfaction because they enable the client to participate more fully in meaningful occupations. Standardized quality-of-life checklists, informal interviews, or other measures of self-report such as the COPM (Law et al., 2005) are all tools that can be used to measure quality of life.

Table 5. Recommendations for Occupational Therapy Interventions for Home Modifications

Modification Type	Recommendation
Home modifications to prevent falls	
Multicomponent interventions (home modifications and other fall prevention interventions) that include occupational therapy to reduce falls	A
Single-component intervention (home modification) including occupational therapy to prevent falls	A
Multicomponent interventions not including occupational therapy to prevent falls	I
Home modifications to improve functional performance	
Home modification interventions to improve function in frail older adults	A
Home modification interventions to improve function for older adults aging with physical disabilities	C
Home modification interventions at discharge for postoperative hip repair	C
Home modification interventions for people with low vision to improve quality of life	C
Intensive, tailored home modification interventions to improve functional performance for community-dwelling people with schizophrenia	C
Caregiving	
Home modification interventions to improve the ability to provide care to others in the home, especially those with dementia	A
Home modification interventions to improve the functional ability of care recipients in the home setting	A
Home modification interventions to reduce caregiver upset for people aging with dementia	C

Note. Criteria for level of evidence and recommendations (A, B, C, I, D) are based on standard language (Agency for Healthcare Research and Quality, 2012). Suggested recommendations are based on the available evidence and content experts' clinical expertise regarding the value of using the intervention in practice. A = There is strong evidence that occupational therapy practitioners should routinely provide the intervention to eligible clients. Good evidence was found that the intervention improves important outcomes and that benefits substantially outweigh harm. B = There is moderate evidence that occupational therapy practitioners should routinely provide the intervention to eligible clients. There is high certainty that the net benefit is moderate or moderate certainty that the net benefit is moderate to substantial. C = There is weak evidence that the intervention can improve outcomes. It is recommended that the intervention be provided selectively on the basis of professional judgment and patient preferences. There is at least moderate certainty that the net benefit is small. I = There is insufficient evidence to determine whether occupational therapy practitioners should be routinely providing the intervention. Evidence that the intervention is effective, is lacking, of poor quality, or conflicting, and the balance of benefit and harm cannot be determined. D = Occupational therapy practitioners are recommended to not provide the intervention to eligible clients. At least fair evidence was found that the intervention is ineffective or that harm outweighs benefits.

Participation

The World Health Organization (2001, p. 10) has defined *participation* as "involvement in a life situation." Home modifications may allow people with a disability to participate in situations that they were previously not able to because of existing barriers in the home setting. For example, an older adult client who uses a wheelchair for mobility was previously not able to access the finished basement of his ranch-style home. However, that is where his adult children and grandchildren stay when they come to visit, and he wanted to be able to be with his grandchildren in that space. The home renovation included the installation of a residential elevator that now allows the client to access the lower level and, more important, be involved in his grandchildren's play. Measurement at the participation level may be completed by using formal assessment tools such as the Activity Card Sort (Baum

& Edwards, 2008) or through informal observation and self-report.

Role Competence

Implementation of modifications may enhance a client's ability to complete the tasks that make up major life roles. For instance, the installation of a side-opening crib may enhance the role of mother for a client who uses a wheelchair for mobility. Likewise, the use of a bedside commode for nighttime toileting needs may increase a caregiver's ability to provide care for his spouse. Role checklists and other measures of self-report can be used to document the extent to which the implementation of home modifications assists a client with the performance of occupations that fulfill a designated life role.

Well-Being

One outcome of the home modification evaluation and intervention may be improved well-being or a sense of contentment and security. Home modifications may lead to improved well-being because the client may experience improved safety and independence at home. The client may also experience reduced fear regarding the need to transition to an alternative living environment. Measures of satisfaction can be used to document the extent to which the home modification process improved the client's sense of well-being and contentment.

Occupational Justice

Occupational justice means having access to and participation in the full range of meaningful and enriching occupations afforded to others (Townsend & Wilcock, 2004). Occupational justice may be considered when monitoring the outcomes of a home modification intervention. The implementation of home modifications may afford a client the opportunity to engage in meaningful occupations that he or she may be deprived of in either the cli-

ent's own home before the modifications or in an institutionalized setting. Similarly, home modifications may increase the length of time that a client is able to live at home and thus the client's access to opportunities and resources that may not be available in other settings. Improved access to the home environment does not simply result in access to the physical features of the home; rather, it may also provide access to desired occupations that a client may not be able to experience elsewhere.

Discontinuation, Discharge Planning, and Follow-Up

Planning for discharge from occupational therapy services should begin during evaluation with consideration of the needs and desires of the client and his or her significant others. Discontinuation of occupational therapy services in the area of home modifications should occur when

- The client achieves his or her established goals through the delivery of home modifications and subsequent education and training in their use;
- The client has achieved maximum benefit from skilled occupational therapy services; or
- Home modifications are no longer needed.

A discharge plan should include regularly scheduled follow-up communication with the client to ensure that the services that were provided continue to meet the client's needs and that no further services are needed.

After the home modifications have been installed, occupational therapists provide follow-up education and training regarding the proper use of the architectural changes, adaptive equipment, and behavioral strategies that were included in the plan. Training and education may occur over one or several occupational therapy intervention sessions. Once the training has been completed and the client is able to demonstrate integration of the home modifications into daily routines and habits, the goals of the intervention should be reviewed. If the identified goals have been achieved and no further goals are established, occupational therapy services should be discontinued.

When a client is receiving home modification interventions within the continuum of acute or post-acute care, the home modifications process may coincide with more than one segment or level of the care continuum. When follow-up education and training cannot be completed before discharge from the client's current level of care, occupational therapists should make a referral to another occupational therapist at the next level of care. For example, an occupational therapist completes a home assessment as part of a plan of care with a client in an inpatient rehabilitation setting. However, the client is discharged from inpatient rehabilitation before the installation of the home modifications. The inpatient rehabilitation therapist should ensure that a referral is made to home health or outpatient therapy so that an occupational therapist can ensure that the home modifications intervention plan is implemented, the client or caregiver receives appropriate training to use the modifications effectively, and targeted outcomes are achieved. The findings of the in-home assessment and the home modification intervention plan should be conveyed to the next provider organization to ensure a smooth care transition.

There are occasions when home modification intervention does not achieve all stated goals. Rather, after all client-centered approaches have been explored, the client may demonstrate improvement in desired occupations, but not to the extent that the client's goals are achieved. For example, a client with hemiparesis has a goal of toileting independently. Through the home modification process, the client-centered home modifications of grab bars, a raised toilet seat, and an adapted flushing mechanism are installed; however, caregiver assistance continues to be needed for safe completion of this task.

In these cases, discontinuation of occupational therapy services may occur even though the client's goals are not achieved. The home modifica-

tions maximize the client's performance of the task while reducing the amount of caregiver assistance needed; however, the goal of independence was not achieved. In this event, discontinuation of occupational therapy services occurs when maximum progress toward the client's goals has been achieved in his or her identified goals.

Finally, discontinuation of occupational therapy for home modifications may occur before the intervention plan is fully implemented. Reasons for discontinuation may include an unanticipated improved level of recovery so that home modifications are no longer needed, a decline in the client's medical status necessitating a move out of the home environment, a change in living arrangement, or a move to another location outside the therapist's or provider's service area. When these unforeseen circumstances arise, occupational therapy services are discontinued. Referral or follow-up may be made to appropriate providers as the situation warrants.

Working With Organizations to Serve People Needing Home Modifications

Occupational therapy practitioners may work with a variety of organizations and businesses involved in the delivery of home modification services. Occupational therapy practitioners may enter into different arrangements or relationships with such organizations. In general, these arrangements are one of three types: (1) referral, (2) consultation, and (3) capacity building.

Referral

In a referral arrangement, the occupational therapy practitioner and the client have a direct relationship. Specifically, the occupational therapy practitioner is working directly with the client whose need for home modifications has been identified through the occupational therapy process. The practitioner makes a referral to one or more organizations to implement some or all the modifications. The organization may be a remodeling business, a nonprofit organization, a branch of local government, or any other business or organization whose services are necessary to execute modifications.

The organization or business is a resource enlisted by the practitioner to implement the interventions identified to achieve specific client outcomes. The organization or business will likely enter into its own formalized relationship with the client. The interventions and outcomes of home modifications are based on the occupational therapy intervention plan and the outcomes jointly agreed on by the practitioner and the client.

In a referral arrangement, the occupational therapy practitioner must obtain the client's permission to share client information with other organizations or businesses. Occupational therapy practitioners are also obligated to disclose to the client any financial relationship that exists between the practitioner and the organizations to which the referral is made (AOTA, 2010).

Consultation

A consultative arrangement is one in which the occupational therapy practitioner provides services on behalf of an organization or business that provides home modifications. Occupational therapy practitioners may serve in a volunteer capacity or may be employed by or otherwise compensated by the organization. Such an arrangement, whether volunteer or compensated, is much like the relationship occupational therapy practitioners have when they are employed or volunteer for any business or organization.

The organization or business establishes a formal agreement with the occupational therapy practitioner to provide consultative services under the auspices of the organization. This formal agreement specifies that the occupational therapy practitioner will use the occupational therapy process as a part of the organization's home modification services.

The formal agreement between the organization and the occupational therapy practitioner will define the practitioner's responsibilities. In general, a formal relationship (reduced to writing as an agreement or contract) also exists between the organization and its service recipient (or client). In most cases, practitioners advise and make recommendations to the organization regarding the modifications to be implemented and the outcomes achievable from such modifications. Practitioners should also recommend and advocate for training in use of the modifications once they are executed if such training is necessary to support the desired outcomes.

In a consultation arrangement, the practitioner and the client have no formalized relationship. The practitioner's relationship with the client is incidental to the organization's relationship with the client. The client's personal information, including to whom it may be disclosed, is governed by the organization's relationship with the client. The findings of the occupational therapy evaluation, as well as the identified goals and interventions, are incorporated into the organization's services to the client. The organization ultimately determines what services will be provided to its client, what modifications will be implemented, and whether training will be provided after the modifications are installed.

Just as in practice with individuals, occupational therapy services being provided under both referral and consultation arrangements are subject to the occupational therapy practice act in the state or jurisdiction in which the modifications are to be implemented. The practice act and any related regulations apply to occupational therapy services, regardless of whether the practitioner is compensated or acting in a volunteer capacity. Such services must be provided under the direction of an occupational therapist. If the state practice act requires a referral from a physician or other medical provider, such a referral must be obtained in accordance with the practice act. It is occupational therapy practitioners' duty to ensure that all occupational therapy services provided are in compliance with the practice act. When occupational therapy services are being provided under the auspices of an organization (consultative arrangement), it is occupational therapy practitioners' responsibility to educate the organization or include language in the service agreement to ensure that the services provided by the practitioner are in compliance with the practice act.

Capacity Building

In a capacity-building arrangement, the occupational therapy practitioner's client is an organization or business. *Capacity building* is defined as actions that improve organizational effectiveness (Blumenthal, 2003). Capacity building is a common concern of nonprofit organizations that may prompt an occupational therapy consultation. Examples of capacity-building outcomes include more effective outreach to service recipients, more effective screening or assessment of service recipient needs, expansion or refinement of the services provided by the organization, establishing or refining knowledge or training of staff and volunteers, and defining or refining the organization's outcome measures.

In a capacity-building arrangement, no direct relationship exists between the occupational therapy practitioner and the organization's service recipients. As part of the collaboration between the occupational therapy practitioner and the organization, the practitioner may be given access to individual or aggregate information about the organization's service recipients. The practitioner may have contact with one or more service recipients. Such access or contact may inform advice given or recommendations made by the practitioner to the organization regarding the services the organization provides or the outcome measures the organization adopts. Because the client is the organization, the occupational therapy practitioner has no direct responsibility for, or control of, the services the organization provides to a given person or population.

Both consultation and capacity building benefit populations that might otherwise not be served by direct occupational therapy services. Tools, services, or service delivery strategies developed in consultation with occupational therapy practitioners can enable an organization to build its capacity and thereby enhance its effectiveness. Case 1 describes how occupational therapy practitioners have consulted with Rebuilding Together, a national nonprofit organization, using evidence-based assessments and practices (see Box 1).

Box 1. Case 1. Example of Occupational Therapy Services to Organizations and Populations

---

Rebuilding Together is a national organization whose mission is "bringing volunteers and communities together to improve the homes and lives of low-income homeowners" (Rebuilding Together, n.d.-b). The organization consists of approximately 200 local affiliates throughout the United States (Rebuilding Together, n.d.-a). For more than a dozen years, Rebuilding Together affiliates and the national Rebuilding Together organization have worked with occupational therapy practitioners to conduct home assessments for their clients.

Occupational therapists have played an important role in providing recommendations for home modifications that will reduce fall risk and enhance function for older adult Rebuilding Together clients. In 2011–2012, Rebuilding Together obtained grant funding from the U.S. Department of Housing and Urban Development for a pilot project involving healthy homes and home safety. Occupational therapists in the three pilot cities participated in a volunteer capacity in providing home assessments, including the In-Home Occupational Therapy Evaluation (HOME FAST); the Safety Assessment of Function and the Environment for Rehabilitation–Health Outcome and Measurement Evaluation, Version 3 (SAFER–HOME v.3); and a nonstandardized occupational therapy assessment.

Capacity building is also a means to address home modification needs in a population served by an organization even if the organization is not directly involved in the delivery of home modifications. For example, an organization that provides home-delivered meals has identified a second aspect of its mission: monitoring and supporting the health and well-being of its service recipients during daily meal delivery. As the organization explores options to enhance its capacity in this area, it recognizes that many of its service recipients have experienced a fall in the home. Reducing the risk of falls supports the well-being of the population served, but it is not clear how the organization can reduce that risk without a complete overhaul of its services. The organization consults with an occupational therapist regarding options to support fall prevention.

The outcome of this collaboration is a falls risk screening designed by the occupational therapist. The screening can be conducted by the volunteers who deliver the meals or can be self-administered by service recipients. As a follow-up to the screening, educational materials specifically selected or designed by the occupational therapist are provided to the service recipients. The materials include information on accessing occupational therapy for an in-home assessment.

To monitor the effectiveness of this new effort, the organization includes an inquiry about falls in the daily monitoring conducted by meal delivery staff. The organization will collect this reported falls data as a measure of the falls experienced by its service population and of the impact of implementing the assessment and follow-up materials.

Best Practices and Summaries of Evidence

This section includes both an overview of specific interventions and findings from the systematic review of occupational therapy for home modifications. A standard process of searching for and reviewing literature related to home modification practice was used and is summarized in Appendix C.

Types of Research Reviewed

The research studies presented here include primarily Level I randomized controlled trials; Level II studies, in which assignment to an intervention or a control group is not randomized (cohort study); and Level III studies, which do not have a control group. In this systematic review, Levels I, II, and III evidence for occupational therapy practice were used to answer a particular research question. All studies identified by the review, including those not specifically described in this section, are summarized and cited in full in the evidence table in Appendix D. Readers are encouraged to read the full articles for more details.

For each area of intervention, consistent results in 2 or more Level I studies were considered as strong evidence, and consistent results in 1 Level I study plus more than 2 lower level studies were considered as moderate evidence (U.S. Preventive Services Task Force, 2012). When only 1 Level II study or consistent results in multiple lower level studies were found, these interventions were rated as having limited evidence (U.S. Preventive Services Task Force, 2012). Finally, inconsistent results among studies were described as having mixed evidence.

Home modifications vary from checklists with preselected hazards to performance-based assessments to assess needs for home modifications. Additionally, the extent to which the intervention is provided varies. A clinician may visit the home one time and leave the client with a list of recommendations or may visit the home over an extended period of time, ensuring modifications are obtained and the client is trained in their use.

Falls Reduction

Consequences from falls can negatively affect a person's ability to successfully age in place. Falls are the leading cause of injury and death for older adults and can significantly reduce the chances for healthy aging. Injuries from falls can make it difficult to get around or live independently, which can have a significant impact on the daily life of older adults (Alexander, Rivara, & Wolf, 1992). People who have experienced a fall are at greater risk for future falls (Stevens, Corso, Finkelstein, & Miller, 2006). Fear of falling is an often unrecognized consequence of falls (Arfken, Lach, Birge, & Miller, 1994), and people who develop a fear of falling may limit their activities, negatively affecting mobility and fitness.

Clemson et al. (2008) developed a rating system for environmental interventions addressing fall prevention on the basis of best practice recommendations. High-quality interventions include 75% of the following criteria:

(a) a comprehensive evaluation process of hazard identification and priority setting taking into account both personal risk and environmental audit, (b) the use of an assessment tool validated for the broad range of potential fall hazards, (c) inclusion of formal or observational evaluation of the functional capacity (physical capacity, behavior, functional vision, habits) of the person within the context of their environment, and (d) provision of adequate follow-up by the health professional and support for adaptations and modifications. (p. 957)

The professional training of the interventionist also plays an important role in the effectiveness of the intervention. According to Clemson et al., occupational therapists have high-level training in evaluating the person and environment.

Sixteen articles in this systematic review addressed the effectiveness of home modifications in reducing falls. Fourteen articles reported on Level I studies (Campbell et al., 2005; Clemson et al., 2004; Close et al., 1999; Cumming et al., 1999; Davison et al., 2005; Hendriks et al., 2008; Huang & Acton, 2004; La Grow et al., 2006; Lin, Wolf, Hwang, Gong, & Chen, 2007; Nikolaus & Bach, 2003; Pardessus et al., 2002; Pighills, Torgerson, Sheldon, Drummond, & Bland, 2011; Tinetti et al., 1999; van Haastregt et al., 2000), and 1 study provided Level III evidence (Plautz, Beck, Selmar, & Radetsky, 1996). Home modifications were provided as both single-component and multicomponent interventions. Overall, the evidence that home modifications provided by occupational therapy reduce falls is strong.

Multicomponent and Single-Component Interventions

Effectiveness of Multicomponent Interventions to Reduce Falls

The multicomponent interventions to reduce falls, including home modifications, exercise, gait training, risk factor education, and medical interventions, modified both intrinsic and extrinsic fall risk factors. These interventions were provided by one or more professionals including occupational therapists, physicians, physical therapists, trained paraprofessionals, and nurses. Owing to the multiple interventions included in multicomponent interventions, determining the impact of the interventions on outcomes is difficult. The variation in the home modification component further complicates understanding these interventions. Of the 15 articles, 9 fall prevention studies included multicomponent interventions combining home modifications with additional fall reduction strategies (Campbell et al., 2005; Clemson et al., 2004; Close et al., 1999; Davison et al., 2005; Hendriks et al., 2008; La Grow et al., 2006; Poulstrup & Jeune, 2000; Tinetti et al., 1999; van Haastregt et al., 2000). On the basis of this research, strong evidence supports multicomponent interventions including home modifications to reduce falls.

Multicomponent interventions including occupational therapists

In combination, 5 Level I studies (Campbell et al., 2005; Clemson et al., 2004; Close et al., 1999; Davison et al., 2005; LaGrow et al., 2006) provided strong evidence for a reduction in falls for older adults participating in multicomponent programs including an occupational therapist. Davison et al. (2005) and Close et al. (1999) provided individualized interventions, including medical, physical therapy, and occupational therapy (Davison et al., 2005) and medical and occupational therapy (Close et al., 1999) for older adults who presented to the emergency department with a fall-related injury. Davison et al. provided a home hazard assessment and plan for removal, and the intervention group had a 36% reduction in falls. Close et al. identified home hazards and provided minor home repair, adapted equipment, and referral for extensive modifications. The risk and rate of falling were lower in the intervention group at 12 months.

Stepping On, a small-group learning program, addresses risk appraisal, exercise, home hazards, community safety, vision, medication management, and planning for fall prevention for older adults with a fall history in the previous 12 months or who are concerned about falling (Clemson et al., 2004). The intervention group had a 31% reduction in falls, with 70% adhering to at least 50% of the home modification recommendations.

Finally, Campbell et al. (2005) and LaGrow et al. (2006) reported results from a single trial comparing a home safety and modification program, exercise program, home modifications and exercise, and social visits for older adults with severe visual impairments. Participants who received the home safety and modifications program had fewer falls (Campbell et al., 2005), and the home safety and modifications group had reduced hazard- and non–hazard-related falls compared with the social visits group (LaGrow et al., 2006).

Multicomponent interventions without occupational therapists

Three studies included multicomponent interventions that did not include occupational therapists. Poulstrup and Jeune (2000) provided written and verbal information to adults ages 65 or older and home assessments to those ages 70 or older using nurses, general practitioners, and home helpers. No significant reduction in fall injury was found between the intervention and control groups. A significant reduction in lower-extremity fractures was found. Tinnetti et al. (1999) provided home-based physical therapy and functional therapy after hip fracture. The functional therapy was completed by a nurse and included task modification, use of adaptive equipment, environmental modifications, psychological interventions, caregiver education, and referrals. No significant difference was seen in falls between groups. Finally, van Haastregt et al. (2000) found no reduction in falls after medical, environmental, and behavioral screening and recommendations completed by nurses. This evidence supports

the unique role of occupational therapy as part of multicomponent fall prevention.

One Level I study (Huang & Acton, 2004) did not report the interventionist's level of training. Huang and Acton (2004) conducted a multicomponent intervention to improve knowledge of medication safety and decrease environmental hazards in the homes of community-dwelling older adults. An environmental hazards and medications checklist was used to assess fall risk factors. The intervention group received three home visits including verbal teaching, individualized brochures, and standardized brochures on fall risk factors concerning environmental hazards and medications. The control group received the standardized fall prevention brochure. At 2 months, falls were reduced and fall self-efficacy was improved for both groups. The short, 2-month follow-up period and lack of information on removal of home hazards make it difficult to interpret the results of this intervention.

Effectiveness of Single-Component Interventions to Reduce Falls

Interventions were considered single component if they targeted changing only the environmental risk factors of falling. The majority of the interventions were provided by occupational therapy and ranged from written recommendations for home hazard removal to individualized assessment of and training in home modification recommendations. Of the 15 articles addressing fall prevention, 6 investigated single-component interventions, providing Level I evidence (Cumming et al., 1999; Lin et al., 2007; Nikolaus & Bach, 2003; Pardessus et al., 2002; Pighills et al., 2011) and Level III evidence (Plautz et al., 1996).

Home Modifications Interventions

Cumming et al. (1999) conducted a comprehensive home assessment by an occupational therapist that assisted with modifications and completed follow-up visits as necessary for community-dwelling older adults. Approximately 50% of the recommendations were completed at 1 year. The intervention was effective only among participants who had a fall history within the 12 months preceding study enrollment.

Nikolaus and Bach (2003) used a team of nurses, physical therapists, and occupational therapists to identify home hazards, prescribe technical aids, and facilitate home modifications for older adults showing functional decline. In the intervention group, 74% made at least one recommended change. The intervention reduced falls by 31%, with adults who completed at least one recommended change experiencing a significant reduction in falls. Additionally, Pardessus et al. (2002) provided one home visit during a hospital stay to identify and recommend changes to reduce home hazards. The level of professional training (physician or occupational therapist) of the intervention provider was unclear. The rate of falls and hospitalization owing to falls was not significantly different from that of the control group. In combination, these studies provide strong evidence for home modification interventions including occupational therapists.

In contrast, Lin et al. (2007) and Pighills et al. (2011) used health professionals other than occupational therapists to complete home modification interventions. Both studies investigated older adults requiring medical attention after a fall. Lin et al.

(2007) used public health workers to assess and remove hazards on the basis of a list of common home hazards. No significant difference in falls was found between groups. Pighills et al. (2011) compared interventions completed by occupational therapists and domiciliary support workers. Both groups completed a training program. The occupational therapists made more recommendations per visit than the support workers and had higher rates of adherence. The occupational therapy group fell significantly less than did the control group. The support worker group did not have significantly different fall rates than the control group.

Summary of Falls Prevention Interventions

The systematic review of the literature found that intensive home modification interventions, when provided by occupational therapists, resulted in a decreased rate and risk of falls among older adults at high risk for falls. Strong evidence was found to support the efficacy of multicomponent interventions that included a home modification component and single-component home modification intervention when delivered by occupational therapists. Please refer to Box 2 for a case example demonstrating the effectiveness of home modifications for reducing falls.

Box 2. Case 2. Home Modifications to Reduce Falls

Mrs. Cook is an 89-year-old African American woman with a history of 5 falls and multiple chronic conditions, including diabetes, diabetic retinopathy, and incontinence. She lives in an urban core in an economically depressed region and is served by the Area Agency on Aging (AAA), which provides home-delivered meals and transportation services. The outpatient occupational therapist received a referral from the AAA for occupational therapy evaluation and intervention to address safety and fall prevention. Her occupational therapy services were funded through Medicare Part B. Evidence suggests Mrs. Cook would benefit from a home modification intervention to remove hazards to reduce her risk of falls. The home modification process must include (1) comprehensive assessment in the home, (2) assistance in obtaining home modifications, and (3) training to safely use the modifications.

(Continued)

Box 2. Case 2. Home Modifications to Reduce Falls *(Cont.)*

Mrs. Cook lives in a 50-unit senior apartment complex. The occupational therapist performed the assessment in Mrs. Cook's home, and the assessment revealed she had overall diminished strength and endurance. She was ambulating in her home with a walker. She had intact tactile sensation. She had scattered scotomas in her visual field assessment. An occupational performance assessment using the Canadian Occupational Performance Measure (Law et al, 2005) indicated Mrs. Cook had difficulty with toilet and shower transfers, difficulty collecting her mail from the community mailbox, and difficulty with laundry (both transporting it to the nearest laundry room in the complex and doing her laundry).

On the basis of the evidence, the occupational therapist selected the Westmead Home Safety Assessment (Clemson, 1997) to identify home hazards that may have an impact on Mrs. Cook's fall risk. The Westmead revealed fall risk factors including a lack of grab bars near the walk-in shower and toilet, a slippery finish on the shower floor, toilet height too low for safe transfer, heavy doors between the apartment and laundry facility, lack of a method to transport clothing to the laundry, and low lighting. Current fall evidence suggested that fear of falling was a significant risk factor for future falls. Given Mrs. Cook's history of previous falls, the occupational therapist evaluated falls self-efficacy using the Falls Efficacy Scale International (Yardley et al., 2005). The scale revealed that Mrs. Cook had an increased fear of falling (score = 29).

In conjunction with Mrs. Cook, the occupational therapist developed an intervention plan to resolve the home hazards and reduce Mrs. Cook's fear of falling.

Problem	Solution	Expected Outcome
Unsafe bathroom transfers because of slippery floor surface in shower, lack of seat, and lack of grab rails	Suction-cup antislip (antimicrobial) mat on the shower floor and a nonslip absorbent bathmat outside the shower door; shower chair and grab bars near shower	Improved transfer safety, improved ability to shower independently
Toilet too low for safe transfer	Portable commode over the toilet or a raised toilet seat with arms to increase height and provide arm support for transfer; alternatively, replace toilet with a comfort-height toilet and toilet safety frame	Improved toilet transfers and independence in toileting
Difficulty moving through home, public spaces, and transporting items	Increased lighting (including night-lights with sensors throughout the unit), wheeled utility cart for laundry	Improved ability to transport laundry to laundry area, functional mobility in apartment and in public spaces between the apartment and laundry facilities

A team including Mrs. Cook, her landlord, her daughter, and the AAA caseworker were aware of and approved the modifications. The therapist worked with the AAA to obtain the modifications and with the senior apartment manager to install grab bars in the apartment. The therapist worked with Mrs. Cook to practice using the modifications. The intervention included 1 session devoted to assessment, 1 for intervention planning with Mrs. Cook and the team, and 3 sessions to practice using the modification. At reevaluation, Mrs. Cook was independent in all ADLs. She reported high satisfaction ($M = 9$) and high performance ($M = 9$) for her ADL goals and demonstrated improved falls self-efficacy on the Falls Efficacy Scale International (score = 20, indicating improved self-efficacy).

Improving Functional Performance

The ability to complete ADLs and IADLs enables people with disabilities to remain in their homes. Estimates have shown that 13.2 million community-dwelling adults receive help completing ADLs and IADLS (LaPlante, Harrington, & Kang, 2002). Approximately 25% of adults ages 62 or older report difficulty completing one or more ADLs (Federal Interagency Forum on Aging-Related Statistics, 2012). Functional decline associated with disability or aging must be matched with environmental supports to prevent unnecessary functional loss (Lawton & Nahemow, 1973). Typical barriers in the homes of older adults include reaching, stairs, and controls that are difficult to manipulate (Mann et al., 1994; Stark, 2001; Steinfeld & Shea, 1993). The prevalence of decreased functional performance and barriers in the home make the role of home modifications to improve function an important consideration.

Sixteen studies included in this systematic review addressed the effectiveness of home modifications in improving functional performance. Ten studies provided Level I evidence (Brunnström et al., 2004; Gitlin, Corcoran, Winter, Boyce, & Hauck, 2001; Gitlin et al., 2006; Hagsten, Svensson, & Gardulf, 2004; Mann, Ottenbacher, Fraas, Tomita, & Granger, 1999; Tinetti et al., 1999; Tomita, Mann, Stanton, Tomita, & Sundar, 2007; Velligan et al., 2008, 2009; Wilson, Mitchell, Kemp, Adkins, & Mann, 2009), 2 provided Level II evidence (Petersson, Kottorp, Bergström, & Lilja, 2009; Petersson, Lilja, Hammel, & Kottorp, 2008), and 4 provided Level III evidence (Fange & Iwarsson, 2005; Gitlin, Miller, & Boyce, 1999; Stark, 2004; Stark et al., 2009). The majority of the study populations were older adults, with the exception of 2 studies (Velligan et al., 2008, 2009). Most of the studies also used occupational therapists as the interventionists, with the exception of 2 (Fänge & Iwarsson, 2005; Tinetti et al., 1999). The focus of the modifications included smart home technology (Tomita et al., 2007), grab bars (Gitlin et al., 1999), individually tailored assessments and interventions (Gitlin et al., 2006; Stark et al., 2009), and delivery as part of a housing program (Fänge & Iwarsson, 2005; Petersson et al., 2009).

On the basis of the results of this research, strong evidence supports home modification interventions to increase functional performance. See Box 3 for a case example of the effectiveness of home modifications for the improvement of functional performance.

Frail Older Adults

Gitlin et al. (2006) evaluated a multicomponent intervention to modify behavioral and environmental factors. The intervention included occupational and physical therapy, providing home modifications and balance and strength training. Home modifications were obtained, and follow-up was provided. The intervention group reported significantly less difficulty with ADLs and IADLs than the control group. Significantly less fear of falling, greater self-efficacy in managing daily activities, greater use of control-oriented strategies, and reduced home hazards were also reported in the intervention group compared with the control group.

Tomita et al. (2007) evaluated the use of smart home technology. Home assessments were completed, and smart home technology was installed. The intervention group had significantly higher cognitive function and rate of independent living 2 years after the intervention. Additionally, the intervention group maintained functional status, whereas the control group demonstrated a significant decline in function.

Stark et al. (2009, 2004) provided Level III evidence for individualized home modifications, education, and follow-up training on the basis of a comprehensive in-home evaluation. Participants' performance and satisfaction with performance significantly improved after the intervention. No signifi-

Box 3. Case 3. Home Modifications to Improve Functional Performance

Linda is a 60-year-old single woman with multiple chronic conditions including arthritis, hypertension, and diabetes. She was in a motor vehicle accident 3 years ago in which she sustained a back injury. Linda recently fell, and her physician suggested she undergo a home safety assessment. Linda continues to work part-time in human resources for an insurance company. She has private insurance through her employer. Linda lives alone with her two pet cats and is an avid bird watcher.

Linda received outpatient occupational therapy in her home to evaluate her ability to perform her daily activities and recommend home modifications to improve safety and function. As part of her occupational therapy services, the occupational therapist conducted a comprehensive assessment of Linda's abilities. The therapist discovered normal vision, hearing, and sensation; limited upper-extremity functional reach (secondary to pain); reduced functional mobility (use of cane for ambulation); and poor balance. Assessment of her occupational performance and the barriers she encountered in her home was conducted using the In-Home Occupational Performance Evaluation (Stark, Somerville, & Morris, 2010). Linda indicated that she had difficulty with daily activities and leisure activities, including doing the laundry, loading the dishwasher, and managing her groceries. She lives in a condominium, which she owns. The occupational therapist consulted with Linda to identify potential solutions to improve her occupational performance in these areas. A set of solutions was identified, and Linda personally paid for them. The condominium association approved the changes to the exterior of her unit so she could enter and exit her exterior door independently.

Problem	Solution	Expected Outcome
Decreased ability to access washer and dryer and transport laundry within the home	Instruction in behavioral strategies of proper body mechanics and lifting techniques to transfer clothes from washer to dryer, rolling cart to transport clothes to and from laundry room	Increased safety and decreased risk of falling during laundry tasks
Decreased ability to reach low dishwasher racks	Installation of a platform to raise the height of the dishwasher	Improved safety and decreased pain when completing kitchen tasks
Difficulty transporting groceries	Use of same wheeled utility cart to transport groceries into the home, rearrangement of pantry so that most commonly used items are located on the middle shelves	Reduced fall risk and increased independence in managing groceries

cant change had occurred in functional independence and performance at 2 years (Stark et al., 2009). Gitlin et al. (1999) also provided Level III evidence evaluating a bathroom modification intervention. An occupational therapist observed bathing and toilet-ing tasks and prescribed modifications. The modifications were installed, and the therapist provided training. A significant improvement was reported for bathing and toilet transfers. Of the participants, 84% reported use of the prescribed equipment.

Two Level I articles provided less intense interventions, showing positive results of reduced declines over time. Wilson et al. (2009) provided people aging with a disability with assistive technology, home modification, and task modification interventions. Both the intervention and the control groups demonstrated a decrease in function, but the intervention group demonstrated slower functional decline. Mann et al. (1999) saw similar results with physically frail older adults who received environmental interventions to improve function; the decline in functional status for the intervention group was significantly less than that in the control group. In combination, these articles provided strong evidence for home modification interventions to improve function in frail older adults.

Significant Functional Impairment

Four articles addressed the impact of home modifications on function for adults aging with physical disabilities. An occupational therapist and an equipment specialist completed a functional home evaluation and made recommendations for home modifications, assistive technology, or behavior modifications (Wilson et al., 2009). If needed, participants were provided with assistance to obtain modifications. Both the intervention and the control groups demonstrated functional decline and an increase in caregiver hours. However, the intervention group demonstrated a slower functional decline than the control group and reported significantly more desired functional changes.

Three articles addressed home modification interventions as part of a housing adaptation program. Participants applied for and received home modifications through housing adaptation grants. Fänge and Iwarsson (2005) found no significant change in ADL scores but saw a decrease in dependence in bathing between 3 months and 9 months after modifications. A significant improvement in perception of the supportiveness of the housing environment occurred. Petersson et al. (2008, 2009) found a significant improvement in self-rated daily activity abilities and reduced difficulty in completing the activity compared with the control group. Time waiting for home modifications had an additional impact on difficulty completing daily activities.

Postoperative Hip Repair

Two articles addressed postoperative home modification interventions among hip fracture patients. Hagsten et al. (2004) investigated individualized ADL training and one home visit to identify necessary environmental modifications completed by occupational therapists during a hospital stay. At 2 months, all participants in the intervention and control groups had regained ADL and IADL abilities. Tinetti et al. (1999) provided home-based functional therapy completed by a nurse, including task modification, use of adaptive equipment, environmental modifications, psychological interventions, caregiver education, and referrals. No significant difference was seen between the intervention and usual-care groups in functional outcomes. High proportions of both groups reported independence in self-care at 6 and 12 months. These results provide limited evidence and indicate a need for additional research to determine the effectiveness of home modification interventions at discharge for postoperative hip repair.

Low Vision

Brunnström et al. (2004) evaluated the effect of home modifications on ADLs for people with low vision, providing Level I evidence. All participants received standard lighting adaptations in the kitchen, bathroom, and hallway, with the intervention group receiving additional task lighting in the living room. Quality of life significantly improved for the intervention group. No change in quality of life or well-being was seen in the control group. The standard lighting adaptations had a significant effect on tasks completed in the working area of the kitchen for both groups. This article provided limited evidence for the effectiveness of home modification interventions to improve quality of life for people with low vision.

Schizophrenia

Velligan et al. (2008, 2009) reported on the efficacy of home modification interventions for community-dwelling people with schizophrenia in a Level I study. The cognitive adaptive training (CAT) group received customized environmental supports based on a comprehensive assessment with weekly home visits, and the generic environmental supports (GES) group received a generic set of environmental supports. In the short term, the CAT and GES groups differed significantly from the control group in social and occupational functioning. Additionally, the CAT group used more supports and was more likely to improve target behaviors than the GES group. Over time, the CAT group demonstrated the most significant improvements, but intervention gains decreased with reduction of session frequency. This Level I study provided positive but limited evidence for the use of an intensive, tailored home modification intervention for community-dwelling people with schizophrenia.

Caregiving for Functional Limitations and Dementia

Caregivers provide unpaid assistance with ADLs and IADLs for people with functional limitations (Donelan et al., 2002). Caregivers deliver more than 85% of assistance, enabling people with disabilities to remain in their personal homes (LaPlante, Kaye, Kang, & Harrington, 2004). People who are under stress are at risk for negative health consequences, including increased cardiovascular and stroke events, depression, and mortality rates (Brotman, Golden, & Wittstein, 2007; Schulz & Beach, 1999). Six articles in the systematic review addressed the effectiveness of home modifications in reducing caregiver assistance. Five articles provided Level I evidence (Dooley & Hinojosa, 2004; Gitlin et al., 2001, 2003;

Graff et al., 2006; Wilson et al., 2009), and 1 article provided Level III evidence (Graff, Vernooij-Dassen, Hoefnagels, Dekker, & de Witte, 2003). All studies used multicomponent approaches with occupational therapists as the interventionists, and most focused on caregivers for people with dementia. See Box 4 for a case example demonstrating the effectiveness of home modifications for reducing negative caregiver outcomes.

Improving Ability to Provide Care for People With Dementia

Four studies addressed the ability to provide care after home modification interventions for people with Alzheimer's disease (AD) or a related disorder (Dooley & Hinojosa, 2004; Gitlin et al., 2003; Graff et al., 2003, 2006). Three articles provided Level I evidence and 1 provided Level III evidence. Gitlin et al. (2003) provided physical and social environmental modification and education for caregivers, resulting in decreased feelings of caregiver burden, fewer days of help from family and friends, and less upset with memory-related problems. Dooley and Hinojosa (2004) also found decreased feelings of caregiver burden after in-home education and environmental adaptations for people with AD and their caregivers. Graff et al. (2003, 2006) increased caregiver sense of competence by educating caregivers on compensatory and environmental strategies. In summary, strong evidence was found that home modification interventions improve the ability to provide care to others in the home, especially those with dementia.

Improving Function for Care Recipients With Dementia

Four studies addressed the effectiveness of home modification interventions to increase function of care recipients with dementia (Dooley & Hinojosa, 2004; Gitlin et al., 2001; Graff et al., 2003, 2006). Of these studies, 3 provided Level I evidence and

---

Box 4. Case 4. Home Modifications to Reduce Negative Caregiver Outcomes

---

Mark is a 46-year-old White man living in a suburban area. He has a BS in accounting, although he has never worked. Mark uses a power chair for mobility and has limited upper-extremity function as the result of cerebral palsy, which was diagnosed at birth. He lives at home with his parents.

Mark's parents are in their late 80s, and both are retired. **Carolyn, his mother,** recently injured her back transferring Mark from his wheelchair to his bed. Her injury required back surgery, and subsequently, she has been receiving home care occupational therapy. She was referred by the Jewish Family Services organization. A physician referral was obtained, and Carolyn's occupational therapy services were funded by Medicare Part B. The occupational therapist completed the In-Home Occupational Performance Evaluation (I–HOPE; Stark, Sommerville, & Morris, 2010) as part of her initial evaluation, and it revealed that caring for Mark was Carolyn's top priority. Barriers to performing the task of caring for Mark were identified as the lack of a mechanical lift to transfer Mark from chair to bed, chair to toilet, and chair to shower. Current evidence has suggested that improving the functional abilities of family members can reduce the demand on caregivers. The family's modest home was given over to the care of their son. He resides in the family den with his medical equipment, hospital bed, and bilevel positive air pressure machine. Space for additional equipment or storage is limited; therefore, an overhead lift was selected.

Working with an overhead lift company, the family, Mark, and the occupational therapist established a plan to install an overhead lift in the bedroom and bathroom. Funding of the lift was identified through a local independent living center administering the state Medicaid waiver program. This funding is targeted to assist people with disabilities to remain living in the community rather than in a nursing home. The program also provides personal attendant services to help Mark perform his daily bathing and dressing, further reducing the physical support required by his mom. After the overhead lift was installed, the occupational therapist provided training and education to Carolyn so that she could perform shower and chair transfers safely using the overhead mechanical lift. Other caregivers, including Mark's father and respite care providers, were also trained to use the lift. Carolyn achieved her goal of independence in assisting Mark with his transfers. She reported a performance score of 5/5 and a satisfaction with performance score of 5/5 on the I–HOPE for the problem of caring for her adult child.

Problem	Solution	Expected Outcome
Difficulty in assisting adult child with chair-to-bed, chair-to-toilet, and chair-to-shower transfers	Installation of a mechanical overhead lift in the bedroom and bathroom, caregiver training to use the lift effectively	Independence in assisting adult child with bed, toilet, and shower transfers

---

1 provided Level III evidence. Graff et al. (2003, 2006) provided interventions targeting both the care provider and the care recipient, resulting in increased function for the care recipient. Gitlin et al. (2003) and Dooley and Hinojosa (2004) provided interventions targeted at the caregiver. Gitlin et al. (2001) provided an environmental skill-building program to educate caregivers of people with dementia on the disease process, environmental effects on behavior and function, problem solving to manipulate the environment to manage caregiving concerns, and generalization to emerging problems. Caregivers in

the intervention group reported significantly less decline in IADL independence for care recipients.

Dooley and Hinojosa (2004) provided written occupational therapy recommendations addressing environmental modifications, caregiver approaches, and community-based assistance for caregivers of people with dementia. The intervention group saw a significant main effect in quality of life (positive affect, activity frequency, and self-care status) for the care recipient. On the basis of this research, the evidence that home modification interventions improve the functional ability of care recipients in the home setting is concluded to be strong.

Reducing Caregiver Hours for People With Early-Onset Disability

One Level I study (Wilson et al., 2009) addressed the effectiveness of a home modification interven-tion to reduce the number of caregiving hours for people aging with early-onset disability. An occupational therapist and equipment specialist provided recommendations for home modifications, assistive technology, or behavior modifications to people aging with a disability. A significant increase in caregiver hours occurred over time for both the intervention and the control groups. No significant difference was reported in caregiving hours between the intervention and control groups. This article provided limited evidence for reduced need for caregiver assistance by people aging with disability and indicates the need for future research in this area.

Implications of the Evidence for Occupational Therapy Research, Education, and Clinical Practice

Summary

Home modifications involve a multistep process that includes a comprehensive evaluation, the development of an intervention plan to reduce identified barriers to occupational performance, facilitation of the procurement of modifications, and follow-up training and education. A systematic review of the literature found strong evidence that home modifications, when provided by occupational therapy practitioners, are effective in improving functional performance, reducing falls or other injuries, and improving the ability to care for others in the home. The evidence indicates that greater outcomes are achieved with increased intensity of home modification assessment, intervention, and follow-up training; it also supports the unique role of occupational therapy practitioners in this area of practice.

The evidence has several implications for occupational therapy researchers, educators, and practitioners. Although the existing literature provides strong support for occupational therapy in home modifications, more research is needed to better understand which components of home modification assessment and intervention are most effective. Occupational therapy educators need to provide entry-level practitioners with the tools needed to practice in the area of home modification, including knowledge and skill in the use of standardized assessment measures, intervention strategies, and research evidence regarding efficacy. Finally, occupational therapy practitioners working with adults in a variety of settings should consider home modification assessment and intervention early in the overall occupational therapy process and ensure that not only assessment but also intervention that includes training and education in the use of home modification strategies is integrated into the occupational therapy intervention plan across the continuum of care.

The goal of occupational therapy in home modifications is to maximize participation in desired occupations in the home setting in a manner that is client centered, occupation based, and grounded in evidence. Participation is maximized when the client is able to integrate the identified home modification solutions into his or her daily habits and routines, thereby improving or sustaining occupational performance. As a result, home modifications, when provided by occupational therapy practitioners, can prevent premature institutionalization and promote health, well-being, and quality of life.

Implications for Research

The findings of the systematic review contribute to the growing body of literature supporting home modification interventions to improve participation, highlighting areas requiring additional occupational therapy research. A consensus conference is needed to develop standards for reporting future research with an operational definition of *home modification interventions*. Areas to address include provider expertise and training, standardized assessments and outcomes, measurement of the magnitude of problems in the home, and length of follow-up periods to create standardized and comparable outcomes across research. On the basis of the results from the systematic review, suggestions for future research are as follows:

- Determine the critical elements of home modification intervention provided by occupational therapy professionals (the "black box" of occupational therapy) that result in improved outcomes compared with other disciplines providing home modifications.
- Determine the intervention intensity and dose of intervention required for successful home modification interventions to improve function and decrease falls.
- Conduct translational research including implementation studies in the United States to guide future policy.
- Conduct single-intervention studies to understand the role home modification plays in reducing the rate and risk of falls. It is difficult to determine the role home modifications play in reducing fall risk when combined with other interventions.
- Investigate the effect of home modification for fall prevention on groups with different diagnoses or health conditions, including dementia, and determine its effectiveness for a range of people.
- Explore the efficacy of environmental modifications to reduce caregiving strain for caregivers and care recipients with a variety of diagnoses influencing functional performance. Develop objective measures to examine the influence of home modifications on caregiver assistance.
- Conduct research using standardized assessments addressing person–environment fit for identifying barriers in the home for functional studies.
- Evaluate the effectiveness of home modifications throughout the continuum of care to increase function and safety in the home.

- Investigate factors that increase adherence to home modification recommendations.

Implications for Education

Entry-level occupational therapy education must address the fundamentals of providing evidence-based home modification intervention. Students should be instructed to provide comprehensive assessment of the person's abilities and the environmental features that influence occupational performance. They should also understand how to conduct a basic task analysis to identify environmental barriers and supports and how to work with a team to procure these supports. Additionally, students should be educated in how to provide training to safely use environmental supports and reestablish habits and routines with home modifications to achieve occupational performance goals. Moreover, curricula should include opportunities to observe and participate in home modification services through fieldwork and other active learning experiences.

Occupational therapy education should also focus on the importance of documenting outcomes to demonstrate the effectiveness of home modification services provided. Students need to understand and articulate the outcomes that can be achieved with home modifications, including reduced caregiver stress, improved functional performance, and reduced risk of falls among older adults. Occupational therapy practitioners must communicate to others the value of the service. Finally, students should understand societal and demographic shifts that will drive the increased need for home modification services, including the client's preference to stay at home rather than move or relocate to a care facility.

Implications for Clinical Practice

The findings of the systematic review identify three outcomes associated with occupational therapy home modifications interventions: (1) improved functional performance, (2) reduced risk of falls, and (3) reduced demands on caregivers. These outcomes are priorities in relation to public sentiment, specifically the expectation to stay active and living in the community through the adult and older adult years. These outcomes are also priorities to policymakers addressing societal health needs and resources. Evidence-based occupational therapy home modification interventions can effectively address needs where public sentiment and public policy converge: supporting health and participation of adults and older adults living at home.

On the basis of the evidence and the growing importance of the associated outcomes, recommendations for clinical practice are as follows:

• Occupational therapy practitioners working with adults and older adults should consider how home modifications can support and sustain outcomes related to functional performance, reducing fall risk and reducing demands on caregivers. This consideration of home modifications should occur throughout the health service continuum, including acute and postacute care, primary care, and community-based practice.

• When an adult or older adult receives acute and postacute care, occupational therapy practitioners across the care continuum should coordinate to ensure that comprehensive intervention is initiated, implemented, and completed. The intervention may thus begin at one phase of care (e.g., inpatient postacute) and be completed at another phase of care (e.g., home health or community-based practice). It is not adequate practice to make a home modification recommendation and expect that the patient will be able to implement the recommendation and achieve the expected result. Effective intervention involves follow-up to ensure that interventions have been implemented and integrated into habits and routines.

• The evidence supports that the basic home modification process—evaluation; intervention, including task analysis conducted with the client in the home environment; implementation of the modifications; and training for their effective use—is entry-level, generalist practice. Opportunities exist within home modifications to develop specialist skills, particularly in the area of complex architectural modifications and advanced adaptive equipment or technologies, but home modification as it is presented in this guideline is not specialist practice.

• Occupational therapy practitioners are encouraged to articulate the outcomes of interventions on the basis of the evidence in their efforts to advocate for more robust and more consistent funding of home modification interventions. Currently, funding sources vary across states and localities. This variation involves the types of modifications covered, the people who may receive such funding (e.g., by income, health condition), and the types of dwellings that may be modified (e.g., single vs. multifamily, owned vs. rented). Both existing and potential funding sources for home modifications are interested in outcomes. Effective advocacy involves implementing evidence-based interventions, achieving the associated outcomes, and documenting or articulating the interventions and outcomes consistent with the evidence.

More specific recommendations based on the findings from the systematic review on home modifications are found in Table 5.

AOTA has developed several mechanisms to support professional growth and continuing competency in home modifications, including continuing education opportunities and community service opportunities. Avenues for obtaining formal recognition as a specialist in home modifications include AOTA's Environmental Modification Specialty Certification, the National Association of Home Builders' Certified Aging in Place Specialist (CAPS) designation, or the University of Southern California's Executive Certificate in Home Modifications.

Appendix A. Preparation and Qualifications of Occupational Therapists and Occupational Therapy Assistants

Who Are Occupational Therapists?

To practice as an occupational therapist, the individual trained in the United States

- Has graduated from an occupational therapy program accredited by the Accreditation Council for Occupational Therapy Education (ACOTE®) or predecessor organizations;
- Has successfully completed a period of supervised fieldwork experience required by the recognized educational institution where the applicant met the academic requirements of an educational program for occupational therapists that is accredited by ACOTE or predecessor organizations;
- Has passed a nationally recognized entry-level examination for occupational therapists; and
- Fulfills state requirements for licensure, certification, or registration.

Educational Programs for the Occupational Therapist

These include the following:

- Biological, physical, social, and behavioral sciences

- Basic tenets of occupational therapy
- Occupational therapy theoretical perspectives
- Screening, evaluation, and referral
- Formulation and implementation of an intervention plan
- Context of service delivery
- Management of occupational therapy services (master's level)
- Leadership and management (doctoral level)
- Scholarship
- Professional ethics, values, and responsibilities.

The fieldwork component of the program is designed to develop competent, entry-level, generalist occupational therapists by providing experience with a variety of clients across the lifespan and in a variety of settings. Fieldwork is integral to the program's curriculum design and includes an in-depth experience in delivering occupational therapy services to clients, focusing on the application of purposeful and meaningful occupation and/or research, administration, and management of occupational therapy services. The fieldwork experience is designed to promote clinical reasoning and reflective practice, to transmit the values and beliefs that enable ethical practice, and to develop professionalism and competence in career responsibilities. Doctoral-level students also must complete a doctoral experiential component designed to develop advanced skills beyond a generalist level.

Who Are Occupational Therapy Assistants?

To practice as an occupational therapy assistant, the individual trained in the United States

- Has graduated from an occupational therapy assistant program accredited by ACOTE or predecessor organizations;
- Has successfully completed a period of supervised fieldwork experience required by the recognized educational institution where the applicant met the academic requirements of an educational program for occupational therapy assistants that is accredited by ACOTE or predecessor organizations;
- Has passed a nationally recognized entry-level examination for occupational therapy assistants; and
- Fulfills state requirements for licensure, certification, or registration.

Educational Programs for the Occupational Therapy Assistant

These include the following:

- Biological, physical, social, and behavioral sciences
- Basic tenets of occupational therapy

- Screening and assessment
- Intervention and implementation
- Context of service delivery
- Assistance in management of occupational therapy services
- Scholarship
- Professional ethics, values, and responsibilities.

The fieldwork component of the program is designed to develop competent, entry-level, generalist occupational therapy assistants by providing experience with a variety of clients across the lifespan and in a variety of settings. Fieldwork is integral to the program's curriculum design and includes an in-depth experience in delivering occupational therapy services to clients, focusing on the application of purposeful and meaningful occupation. The fieldwork experience is designed to promote clinical reasoning appropriate to the occupational therapy assistant role, to transmit the values and beliefs that enable ethical practice, and to develop professionalism and competence in career responsibilities.

Regulation of Occupational Therapy Practice

All occupational therapists and occupational therapy assistants must practice under federal and state law. Currently, 50 states, the District of Columbia, Puerto Rico, and Guam have enacted laws regulating the practice of occupational therapy.

Note. The majority of this information is taken from the *2011 Accreditation Council for Occupational Therapy Education (ACOTE®) Standards* (ACOTE, 2012).

Appendix B. Selected *CPT*^{TM} Codes for Occupational Therapy for Home Modifications

The following chart can guide occupational therapists in making clinically appropriate decisions in selecting the most relevant *CPT*™ code to describe occupational therapy evaluation and interventions related to providing home modifica- tions for older adults. Occupational therapy practitioners should use the most appropriate code from the current *CPT* manual on the basis of specific services provided, individual patient goals, payer coding and billing policy, and common usage.

Examples of Occupational Therapy Evaluation and Intervention	Suggested *CPT* Code(s)
Evaluation	
Comprises the initial evaluation of the older adult's status and performance in areas of occupation, performance skills, performance patterns, context and environment, activity demands, and client factors. • Functional evaluation using standardized assessment (e.g., I–HOPE) • Evaluation of client factors (i.e., strength, range of motion, cognition, vision, sensation and perception, and/or psychosocial factors) • Using non-standardized assessment methods such as observation of the client performing tasks within their home environment • Gather data from various other sources (e.g., medical record, occupational profile, interview, caregivers, significant others) • Develop individual goals to address the misfit between the client and their home environment.	**97003**—Occupational therapy evaluation
Formal reassessment of changes in performance due to changes in status, diagnosis, or if intervention plans needs significant revisions. • Re-assessment of the fit between the client and their home environment usually after a change in client status, using standardized and non-standardized assessments.	**97004**—Occupational therapy reevaluation

(Continued)

Examples of Occupational Therapy Evaluation and Intervention	Suggested *CPT* Code(s)
• Administer, interpret, and report findings from assistive technology assessment to identify technology to improve a client's ability to perform tasks within the home environment. *Example:* assess suitability of a custom or commercially available home/environmental control system.	**97755**—Assistive technology assessment (e.g., to restore, augment or compensate for existing function, optimize functional tasks and/or maximize environmental accessibility), direct one-on-one contact by provider, with written report, each 15 minutes
• Participate in a medical team conference as part of an evaluation team whereby the team discusses the evaluation findings and recommendations with a client and his/her family.	**99366**—Medical team conference with interdisciplinary team of health care professionals, face-to-face with patient and/or family, 30 minutes or more, participation by non-physician qualified health care professional
• Participate in a medical team conference as part of evaluation team whereby the team reviews evaluation findings and recommendations prior to meeting with a client and his/her family.	**99368**—Medical team conference with interdisciplinary team of health care professionals, patient and/or family not present, 30 minutes or more; participation by non-physician qualified health care professional
Intervention	
• Develop compensatory methods to perform meal preparation activities using a mobility aid. • Train in methods of adapting bathroom, toilet transfer routine and habit to improve safety and independence in toileting using raised toilet seat with arms. • Train in methods of safe use of renovated walk-in shower. • Train client in the ability to direct a caregiver to perform tasks within the home environment.	**97535**—Self care/home management training (e.g., activities of daily living (ADL) and compensatory training, meal preparation, safety procedures, and instructions in use of assistive technology devices/adaptive equipment), direct one-on-one contact by provider, each 15 minutes
• Train client in the use of modifications or behavioral strategies for community mobility, the care for others, financial management, shopping, or work tasks.	**97537**—Community/work reintegration training (e.g., shopping, transportation, money management, avocational activities and/or work environment/modification analysis, work task analysis, use of assistive technology device/adaptive equipment), direct one-on-one contact by provider, each 15 minutes
• Training in controlling/maneuvering a wheelchair in a newly redesigned space or in relation to an access device (e.g., lift, elevator or ramp).	**97542**—Wheelchair management/propulsion training, each 15 minutes

Note. Not all payers will reimburse for all codes. For example, medical team conferences are not billable to Medicare, but may be useful for reporting productivity. Codes shown refer to *CPT* 2014 (American Medical Association, 2013) and do not represent all of the possible codes that may be used in occupational therapy evaluation and intervention. Refer to *CPT* 2014 for the complete list of available codes. *CPT* codes are updated annually and become effective January 1. *CPT*^TM is a trademark of the American Medical Association. *Current Procedural Terminology* five-digit codes, two-digit codes, modifiers, and descriptions only are copyrighted © by the American Medical Association. All rights reserved.

Appendix C.
Evidence-Based Practice

Occupational therapists and occupational therapy assistants, as do many health care professionals facing the demands of payers, regulators, and consumers, increasingly have to demonstrate clinical effectiveness. In addition, they are eager to provide services that are client centered, supported by evidence, and delivered in an efficient and cost-effective manner. Over the past 20 years, evidence-based practice (EBP) has been advocated widely as one approach to effective health care delivery.

Since 1998, the American Occupational Therapy Association (AOTA) has instituted a series of EBP projects to assist members with meeting the challenge of finding and reviewing the literature to identify evidence and, in turn, use this evidence to inform practice (Lieberman & Scheer, 2002). Following the evidence-based philosophy of Sackett, Rosenberg, Muir Gray, Haynes, and Richardson (1996), AOTA's projects are based on the principle that the EBP of occupational therapy relies on the integration of information from three sources: (1) clinical experience and reasoning, (2) preferences of clients and their families, and (3) findings from the best available research.

A major focus of AOTA's EBP projects is an ongoing program of systematic review of multidisciplinary scientific literature, using focused questions and standardized procedures to identify practice-relevant evidence and discuss its implications for practice, education, and research. An evidence-based perspective is founded on the assumption that scientific evidence of the effectiveness of occupational therapy intervention can be judged to be more or less strong and valid according to a hierarchy of research

designs, an assessment of the quality of the research, or both. AOTA uses standards of evidence modeled on those developed in evidence-based medicine. This model standardizes and ranks the value of scientific evidence for biomedical practice using the grading system based on the work of Sackett et al. (1996) and presented in Table C1. In this system, the highest level of evidence, *Level I,* includes systematic reviews of the literature, meta-analyses, and randomized controlled trials (RCTs). In RCTs, participants are randomly allocated to either an intervention or a control group, and the outcomes of both groups are compared. Other levels of evidence include *Level II* studies, in which assignment to a treatment or a control group is not randomized (cohort study); *Level III* studies, which do not have a control group; *Level IV* studies, which use a single-case experimental design, sometimes reported over several participants; and *Level V* studies, which are case reports and expert opinion that include narrative literature reviews and consensus statements.

The systematic review of home modifications was supported by AOTA as part of the EBP Project. AOTA is committed to supporting the role of occupational therapy in this area of practice on the basis of the importance to older adults of aging in place and an interest in updating the *Occupational Therapy Practice Guidelines for Home Modification* (Siebert, 2005). The systematic review was also developed on basis of the need for occupational therapy practitioners to have access to the results of the latest and best available literature to support intervention within the scope of occupational therapy practice.

Table C.1. Levels of Evidence for Occupational Therapy Outcomes Research

Evidence Level	Definition
I	Systematic reviews, meta-analyses, randomized controlled trials
II	Two groups, nonrandomized studies (e.g., cohort, case control)
III	One group, nonrandomized (e.g., before and after, pretest and posttest)
IV	Descriptive studies that include analysis of outcomes (e.g., single-subject design, case series)
V	Case reports and expert opinion that include narrative literature reviews and consensus statements

Source. From "Evidence-Based Medicine: What It Is and What It Isn't," by D. L. Sackett, W. M. Rosenberg, J. A. Muir Gray, R. B. Haynes, & W. S. Richardson, 1996, *British Medical Journal, 312,* pp. 71–72. Copyright © 1996 by the British Medical Association. Adapted with permission.

One focused question served as the basis for the systematic review: What is the evidence for the effectiveness of home modification interventions within the scope of occupational therapy for adults and older adults to participate in areas of occupation in the home and community? This question was reviewed by the review author, an advisory group of experts in the field, AOTA staff, and the methodology consultant to the AOTA EBP Project. The areas of occupation include activities of daily living (ADLs), instrumental activities of daily living (IADLs), work, education, leisure, and social participation.

Method

Search terms for the reviews were developed by the methodology consultant to the AOTA EBP Project and AOTA staff in consultation with the review author and reviewed by the advisory group. The search terms were developed not only to capture pertinent articles but also to make sure that the terms relevant to the specific thesaurus of each database were included. Table C2 lists the search terms related to the population and intervention included in the systematic review. A medical research librarian with experience in completing systematic review searches conducted all searches and confirmed and improved the search strategies.

Databases and sites searched included Medline, PsycINFO, CINAHL, AgeLine, OTseeker, and Scopus. In addition, consolidated information sources, such as the Cochrane Database of Systematic Reviews, were included in the search. These databases are peer-reviewed summaries of journal articles and provide a system for clinicians and scientists to conduct evidence-based reviews of selected clinical questions and topics. Moreover, reference lists from articles included in the systematic reviews were examined for potential articles, and selected journals were hand searched to ensure that all appropriate articles were included.

Table C.2. Search Strategy for Systematic Review on Home Modifications

Category	Key Search Terms
Population	Limited to adult and older adult
Intervention	Accessible design, built environment, environment design, environmental barriers, environmental hazard, environmental modification, environmental supports, home adaptation, home assessment, home hazards, home modification, home office, home repair, home safety, home safety equipment, housing adaptation, housing for the elderly, person–environment fit, universal design

Inclusion and exclusion criteria are critical to the systematic review process because they provide the structure for the quality, type, and years of publication of the literature incorporated into a review. The systematic review was limited to peer-reviewed scientific literature published in English. The intervention approaches examined were within the scope of practice of occupational therapy. The literature included in the review was published between 1990 and July 2011 and included study participants ages 18 years or older with health conditions that affected function. Studies included in the review are Levels I, II, and III evidence. The review excluded data from presentations, conference proceedings, non–peer-reviewed research literature, dissertations, and theses.

A total of 6,762 citations and abstracts were included in the review. The first author of this practice guideline completed the first step of eliminating references on the basis of citation and abstract. The systematic review was carried out as academic partnerships in which an academic faculty member worked with two graduate students. The review teams completed the next step of eliminating references on the basis of citations and abstracts. The full-text versions of potential articles were retrieved, and the review team determined final inclusion in the review on the basis of predetermined inclusion and exclusion criteria.

A total of 35 articles were included in the final review. The review included 26 Level I studies, 3 Level II studies, and 6 Level III studies. The teams working on the focused question reviewed the articles according to their quality (scientific rigor and lack of bias) and levels of evidence. Each article included in the review was then abstracted using an evidence table that provides a summary of the methods and findings of the article and an appraisal of the strengths and weaknesses of the study on the basis of design and methodology. AOTA staff and the EBP Project consultant reviewed the evidence table to ensure quality control. All studies are summarized in full in the evidence table in Appendix D.

Limitations of the studies incorporated into the review may include small sample sizes, lack of blinding, a high rate of attrition, and limited details on the intervention provided in a given study. Also, in a multicomponent treatment intervention, it is difficult to separate the role of home modification. In several studies there is lack of a control group and lack of randomization. In addition, contamination may have taken place in several studies, as a similar intervention may have been inadvertently provided to the control group.

Appendix D.
Evidence Table

Author/Year	Study Objectives	Level/Design/Participants	Intervention and Outcome Measures	Results	Study Limitations
Brunnström, Sörensen, Alsterstad, & Sjöstrand (2004)	To evaluate the effect of light adjustment on ADLs and to determine whether additional task lighting in the living room reading area affected QoL	Level I RCT $N = 46$ adults with low vision (M age = 76 yr, range = 20–90 yr); $n = 24$ lighting intervention, $n = 22$ control. 12 participants had macular degeneration (dry form), 16 had macular degeneration (wet form), 2 had retinitis pigmentosa, 5 had glaucoma, and 11 had other diagnoses.	*Intervention* All participants received lighting adaptations in the kitchen, bathroom, and hallway. The intervention group received adaptations plus an additional intervention of improved task lighting in the reading area of the living room. *Outcome Measures* Interview about performance of ADLs and QoL.	The QoL for the intervention group improved significantly; the control group had no change in QoL or well-being. The effect of the basic lighting adaptation in kitchen, hall, and bathroom on ADLs for both groups was significant for tasks carried out on the work surface in the kitchen.	Participants were recruited from a low vision clinic. The primary endpoint was not assessed using standardized assessments (ADLs and QoL). Differences between groups on demographic characteristics not available.
http://dx.doi.org/10.1093/ageing/afi053					
Campbell et al. (2005)	To assess the efficacy and cost-effectiveness of a multicomponent intervention (including home safety and a home exercise program) to reduce falls and injuries in older adults with low vision	Level I RCT $N = 391$ older adults ages ≥75 yr with low vision (M age = 83.6 yr); $n = 100$ home safety and modifications only (M age = 83.1 yr), $n = 97$ Otago (home-based) exercise program only (M age = 83.4 yr), $n = 98$ both home modifications and Otago exercise (M age = 83.8 yr), $n = 96$ social visit control (M age = 84.0 yr).	*Intervention* Home safety program included a home safety checklist with referral or recommendations to reduce home hazards by an OT. 90% reported complying partially or completely with 1 or more of the home modification recommendations. The exercise program included a year-long modified exercise program with vitamin D supplementation. Social visits included 2 60-min home visits. *Outcome Measures* Falls and injuries (self-report).	There were 41% fewer falls in the participants of the home safety program compared with those who did not receive the program. No significant difference was found in the reduction of falls at home compared with those away from the home environment. The home safety program cost $432 per fall prevented.	The length of time living with a visual impairment varied significantly. There was low adherence to the home exercise program in this group possibly owing to lack of screening for ability to participate in exercise programs.
http://dx.doi.org/10.1136/bmj.38601.447731.55					

(Continued)

Table D1. Home Modification Interventions for Adults and Older Adults (*Cont.*)

Author/ Year	Study Objectives	Level/Design/ Participants	Intervention and Outcome Measures	Results	Study Limitations
Clemson et al. (2004)	To determine whether Stepping On is effective in reducing falls in at-risk people living at home	Level I RCT N = 310 community residents ages ≥70 yr with a fall history in the previous 12 mo or who were concerned about falling; n = 157 Stepping On program (74% women, M age = 78.31 yr), n = 153 control (74% women, M age = 78.47 yr).	*Intervention* Stepping On, a multifaceted community-based program led by an OT using small-group learning with follow-up home visit and booster session. Stepping On includes a home hazard removal component. Session topics included risk appraisal, exercises, home hazards, community safety and footwear, vision and falls, medication management, and plan ahead. *Outcome Measures* Falls (self-report).	Intervention group had 31% reduction in falls. 70% of participants adhered to at least 50% of home modification recommendations.	There was a difference in contact time between intervention group and control group. Home modifications were part of a multi-component treatment intervention. Individual effect of home modifications in reducing fall risk is unknown for this multicomponent intervention.

http://dx.doi.org/10.1111/j.1532-5415.2004.52411.x

Close et al. (1999)	To determine whether OT assessment and intervention can decrease rate of falls over a 12-month follow-up period	Level I RCT N = 397 adults ages ≥65 yr living in the community who presented to the emergency department with a fall (M age = 78.2 yr); n = 184 medical and OT assessment (M age = 78.9 yr), n = 213 control (M age = 77.3 yr).	*Intervention* Treatment included OT assessment in the home to identify and remove environmental hazards, safety education, minor home repair, adapted equipment, and referral for extensive modifications. *Outcome Measures* Falls (self-report via mailed follow-up) at 8 and 12 mo. Barthel Index for ADL/IADL performance.	Risk of falling and rate of falling were lower in the intervention group than in the control group in the 12-mo follow-up period. Both groups experienced a reduction in Barthel scores over time; however, the intervention group had less of a decline.	A high rate of attrition. Limited description of the OT intervention. No objective observation of compliance with recommendations; mailed follow-up only.

(Continued)

Table D1. Home Modification Interventions for Adults and Older Adults *(Cont.)*

Author/ Year	Study Objectives	Level/Design/ Participants	Intervention and Outcome Measures	Results	Study Limitations
Cumming et al. (1999)	To determine whether OT home visits to remove environmental hazards reduce the risk of falls	Level I RCT $N = 530$ community-dwelling adults ages ≥65 yr (M age = 77 yr); $n =$ 264 OT group (M age = 76.4 yr), $n =$ 266 control (M age = 77.2 yr).	*Intervention* Home visit conducted by an occupational therapist. Treatment included comprehensive assessment of person and home and facilitation of home hazard removal. Approximately 50% of recommended home modifications were in place at 12 mo. Control received no home visit. *Outcome Measures* Falls (self-report).	The intervention was effective only among participants ($n = 206$) who reported having had 1 or more falls during the year before recruitment into the study.	No home visit for control group. No way to determine effect of social visit on the outcome. Insufficient sample size to detect an effect for the entire cohort. High rate of refusal for home visit. Total attrition, including death, was 33%.
Davison, Bond, Dawson, Steen, & Kenny (2005)	To determine whether multifactorial, multi-disciplinary intervention (including home modification) reduces falls among recurrent fallers attending accident and emergency departments	Level I RCT $N = 313$ cognitively intact adults ages ≥65 yr who presented to accident and emergency with a fall or fall-related injury and 1 additional fall in the preceding yr; $n = 159$ intervention (M age = 77 yr), $n = 154$ control (M age = 77 yr).	*Intervention* Multifactorial, multidisciplinary intervention targeting fall risk factors including medical, PT, and OT assessment and intervention. OT provided a home hazard assessment and plan for removal. Control group received usual care. *Outcome Measures* Self-reported falls and fear of falling (fall diary); injury rates, fall-related hospital admissions, and mortality.	The intervention group had 36% fewer falls. No difference was found in the risk of fall-related hospital admissions between treatment and intervention groups.	Fall risk factors were not assessed in the control group, making interpretability of the findings difficult. Individual effect of home modifications in reducing fall risk is unknown in this multicomponent intervention. There was bias in the control group because 21% received specialist falls assessment during day hospital physiotherapy, which may have affected the control group outcomes.

http://dx.doi.org/10.1093/ageing/afi053

(Continued)

Table D1. Home Modification Interventions for Adults and Older Adults *(Cont.)*

Author/ Year	Study Objectives	Level/Design/ Participants	Intervention and Outcome Measures	Results	Study Limitations
Dooley & Hinojosa (2004)	To determine whether individualized OT assessment and recommendations for environmental modifications, caregiver strategies, and community-based services improve QoL among community-dwelling people with AD and reduce the burden of their caregivers	Level I RCT *N* = 40 community-dwelling participants in mild-to-moderate stages of AD (*M* age = 77.08 yr) and their caregivers (80% women).	*Intervention* In-home assessment and treatment plan including education and environmental adaptation were provided to person with AD and his or her caregiver. The control group was mailed a written treatment plan (the intervention) at the completion of study follow-up. *Outcome Measures* Caregiver-reported scores on the Affect and Activity Limitation–Alzheimer's Disease Assessment (AAL–AD) and Zarit Burden Interview (ZBI).	A significant main effect was found for caregiver burden, positive affect, activity frequency, and self-care status of the treatment group. Caregivers followed 65.1% of the strategies recommended by the occupational therapist either sometimes or often.	No descriptive data provided by group status. No descriptive information provided for caregivers. Participants were followed for 1 mo. The long-term effects of the treatment are unknown. A single interventionist provided treatment. Treatment recommendations only were provided. No implementation (e.g., facilitating home modification) was provided.

http://dx.doi.org/10.5014/ajot.58.5.561

Fänge & Iwarsson (2005)	To determine the longitudinal changes in ADL performance of adults who receive home modifications (Swedish housing adaptation grants)	Level III Longitudinal; before and after *N* = 131 community-dwelling adults ages ≥18 yr with 1 or more functional limitation who were being considered for housing adaptation grants (88 women, 43 men; age range = 24–93, *M* age = 71 yr).	*Intervention* Housing adaptation grants administered by community-based occupational therapists. Participants were assessed before, 2–3 mo after, and 8–9 mo after housing modification. *Outcome Measures* ADL Staircase, Revised Version; Usability in My Home Instrument (environmental impact on performance of ADL/IADL).	No significant change in total ADL scores at any time point relative to baseline. Decrease in dependence in bathing between Time 2 and Time 3. Client perception of the supportiveness of their housing environment of daily activities increased significantly at Time 2 compared with Time 1. Statistically significant improvements in client perception of the supportiveness of housing environment on personal and social aspects between Time 2 and Time 3.	Other interventions may have been implemented. Housing adaptations may only be useful for a small amount of time owing to decline. No training to use the home modifications was provided. The intervention did not plan for future functional abilities or decline.

http://dx.doi.org/10.5014/ajot.59.3.296

(Continued)

Table D1. Home Modification Interventions for Adults and Older Adults (*Cont.*)

Author/ Year	Study Objectives	Level/Design/ Participants	Intervention and Outcome Measures	Results	Study Limitations
Gitlin, Corcoran, Winter, Boyce, & Hauck (2001)	To determine short-term effects of a home environmental intervention on caregivers and dementia patients	Level I RCT *N* = 171 primary caregivers living with a family member with AD or a related disorder with reported dependence in at least 2 ADLs, reporting difficulty managing ADLs or IADLs or a dementia-related behavior (*M* age = 61 yr, age range = 23–92); *n* = 93 intervention (*M* age = 59.7 yr), *n* = 78 control (*M* age = 61.4 yr).	*Intervention* A multicomponent program led by an occupational therapist included 5 90-min home visits to address physical and social environmental modifications and provide education on the impact of the environment on dementia-related behaviors. The intervention group participated in an average of 4 sessions; 75% of recommendations were implemented. Control group received usual care. *Outcome Measures* Memory and Behavior Problems Checklist, ADL/IADL dependence (FIM™), self-efficacy, upset.	Caregivers in the intervention group reported less decline in IADL dependence in the person with dementia than did control group caregivers at 3-mo posttest. Intervention spouses reported reduced upset. Intervention women reported enhanced self-efficacy in managing behaviors. Intervention women and minorities reported enhanced self-efficacy in managing functional dependency.	Inclusion of groups that did not benefit from the intervention may have diluted the main effects. Intervention effects examined at 1 time point immediately after the intervention; caregivers may need more time to practice strategies. A high dose and level of intensity may be needed. Caregivers may not have had enough time to practice strategies with the study protocol. Adaptive equipment recommendations were not described.

http://dx.doi.org/10.1093/geront/41.1.4

(Continued)

Table D1. Home Modification Interventions for Adults and Older Adults (Cont.)

Author/Year	Study Objectives	Level/Design/Participants	Intervention and Outcome Measures	Results	Study Limitations
Gitlin, Miller, & Boyce (1999)	To evaluate a bathroom modification program for non–home owners A 2-phase study that included (1) OT evaluation bathroom modifications over 2 visits and (2) telephone survey to examine adherence to bathroom modification recommendations	Level III Pretest–posttest *Phase 1:* $N = 34$ participant ages ≥70 yr with 3 or more chronic conditions or a diagnosis of stroke, hip fracture, amputation, balance difficulties, or rheumatoid arthritis (M age = 76 yr, 85.3% women). *Phase 2:* $N = 75$ clients who had received equipment within 3 months of telephone contact.	*Intervention* Occupational therapist observed bathing and toileting tasks, prescribed and had bathroom equipment installed, and provided training to safely use the equipment. *Outcome Measures* Self-reported adherence and level of independence performing bathing and toileting.	Clients who received OT intervention reported significant improvement in bathing and toilet transfers. Clients reported high adherence (84%) to using equipment, and 65% reported difficulty with the equipment (vendor or safety related).	Nonstandardized outcome measures. Pretest–posttest comparison of self-care status between the OT group and non–OT group was not possible. Unable to examine ADL difficulties for the clients who did not receive OT evaluation. Pretest and posttest assessments and instruction conducted by the same therapist. Unable to differentiate whether improvements in self-care resulted from equipment, OT, or the combination of both OT and equipment.

(Continued)

Table D1. Home Modification Interventions for Adults and Older Adults *(Cont.)*

Author/ Year	Study Objectives	Level/Design/ Participants	Intervention and Outcome Measures	Results	Study Limitations
Gitlin et al. (2003)	To examine 6-mo effects of the Environmental Skill-Building Program (ESP) on caregiver well-being and care recipient functioning and whether effects vary by caregiver race, gender, or relationship	Level I RCT $N = 190$ primary caregivers living with a community-residing person with AD or related disorder; care recipient has a minimum of 1 limitation in ADLs or 2 dependencies in IADLs (M age = 60.5 yr); $n = 89$ ESP (M age = 60.4 yr), $n = 101$ control (M age = 60.5 yr).	*Intervention* An OT provided 5 90-min home visits and 1 30-min phone contact to educate caregivers about dementia and the impact of home environments, instruction in problem solving and developing effective approaches to manage caregiving concerns, manipulating the physical and social environment, implementation of environmental strategies, and generalization of strategies to emerging problems. *Outcome Measures* *Person with AD:* modified FIM; Revised Memory and Behavior Problem Checklist (RMBPC). *Caregiver:* Caregiver reaction (upset) scales, Caregiving Mastery Index (CMI), Task Management Strategy Index (TMSI).	At 6 mo, the treatment did not significantly change hours helping with IADLs, upset with providing ADL/IADL assistance, and perceived change in somatic symptoms. No statistically significant treatment effects were found for outcome measures related to care recipient functioning. Caregivers reported using significantly less help from family and friends with ADL activities. Women showed a significant reduction in the number of days receiving help with ADLs compared with control group women. Men reported a significant reduction in time spent caregiving compared with control group. Women showed significant improvement in their ability to manage caregiving.	Unequal social attention from a health professional between groups. Individual effect of home modifications in reducing the amount of help caregiver needed or ability to manage caregiving is unknown for this multicomponent intervention.

http://dx.doi.org/10.1093/geront/43.4.532

(Continued)

Table D1. Home Modification Interventions for Adults and Older Adults *(Cont.)*

Author/ Year	Study Objectives	Level/Design/ Participants	Intervention and Outcome Measures	Results	Study Limitations
Gitlin et al. (2006)	To evaluate a multi-component home-based intervention designed to reduce difficulties in performing everyday tasks in community-dwelling people by modifying behavioral and environmental contributors to functional decline	Level I RCT $N = 319$ urban-dwelling older adults reporting difficulty with 1 or more ADLs (M age = 79 yr); $n = 160$ intervention (M age = 79.5 yr), $n = 159$ control (M age = 78.5 yr).	*Intervention* OT (4 90-min sessions, 1 20-min telephone contact) and PT (1 90-min session) home visits over 6 mo to provide home modifications and training; instruction in problem-solving strategies, energy conservation, and fall recovery techniques; and balance and muscle strength training. Three follow-up telephone calls were made by the OT over an additional 6 mo, and a final home visit was conducted. *Control:* No intervention contact. *Outcome Measures* Self-report measures of functional difficulties with ambulation, IADL, ADL, use of adaptive strategies, presence of home hazards.	At 6 mo, the intervention group reported significantly less difficulty with IADLs and ADLs than controls. The greatest benefits occurred in bathing and toileting. Significantly less fear of falling, greater self-efficacy in managing daily activities, greater use of control-oriented strategies, and reduced home hazards were reported in the intervention group. Average cost for equipment and home modifications was $439.	No-treatment control group. Lack of objective performance; self-report of primary outcomes. Unclear whether 1 intervention component was more effective than other components. Individual effect of home modifications in improving functional abilities is unknown for this multicomponent intervention.

http://dx.doi.org/10.1111/j.1532-5415.2006.00703.x

Author/ Year	Study Objectives	Level/Design/ Participants	Intervention and Outcome Measures	Results	Study Limitations
Graff, Vernooij-Dassen, Hoefnagels, Dekker, & de Witte (2003)	To explore the effects of OT on the performance of daily activities by older people with cognitive impairments and on the sense of competence of their primary caregivers	Level III Single-group design (pretest–posttest) $N = 12$ older adults with mild-to-moderate cognitive impairment (M age = 79.9 yr) and their primary caregiver (M age = 56.6 yr).	*Intervention* OT treatments over 7 wk: during a hospital visit (4 treatment sessions) and in home (10 visits) addressing education, problem solving, training in effective coping strategies, and practical and emotional support in how to deal with the cognitive problems of their relatives. *Outcome Measures* Assessment of Motor and Process Skills (AMPS), Interview of Deterioration of Daily Activities in Dementia (IDDD), Canadian Occupational Performance Measure (COPM).	Motor and process skills increased significantly and the need for assistance performing daily activities decreased significantly at 7 wk. Sense of competence in caregivers significantly improved. Self-perception and satisfaction in occupational performance significantly improved for the participants with cognitive impairments.	Possible influence from other interventions or medication. OT treatment was based on environmental and psychosocial approach. The extent of environmental modifications was not reported.

(Continued)

Table D1. Home Modification Interventions for Adults and Older Adults (*Cont.*)

Author/ Year	Study Objectives	Level/Design/ Participants	Intervention and Outcome Measures	Results	Study Limitations
Graff et al. (2006)	To determine the effectiveness of community-based OT on the daily functioning of patients with dementia and on the sense of competence felt by their primary caregivers	Level I Single-blind RCT $N = 135$ individuals ages ≥ 65 yr with mild-to-moderate dementia living in the community; $n = 68$ OT group (M age = 79.1 yr, caregiver M age = 66.0), $n = 67$ control (patient M age = 77.1 yr, caregiver M age = 61.3 yr).	*Intervention* Treatment provided by OT included 10 1-hr sessions over 5 wk to identify potential targets for intervention and to instruct participants in how to use compensatory and environmental strategies. Caregivers were trained to use effective supervision, problem-solving, and coping strategies. *Outcome Measures* AMPS, IDDD, Sense of Competence questionnaire.	Participants who received OT showed significant improvements in daily life functioning at 6 wk and 3 mo. Primary caregivers felt significantly more competent. Caregivers' sense of competence was significantly better at 12 wk.	Possible bias because patients and caregivers knew the therapy they received. Interventionists were not blind to allocation. Sample likely not representative of all people with dementia (recruited from a single outpatient clinic). No details provided on the environmental strategies implemented. Individual effect of home modifications in improving functioning and improving self-efficacy with caregiving is unknown for this multicomponent intervention.

http://dx.doi.org/10.1136/bmj.39001.688843.BE

(Continued)

Table D1. Home Modification Interventions for Adults and Older Adults (*Cont.*)

Author/ Year	Study Objectives	Level/Design/ Participants	Intervention and Outcome Measures	Results	Study Limitations
Hagsten, Svensson, & Gardulf (2004)	To determine the effects of an early, individualized, post-operative OT training program among hip fracture patients	Level I RCT *N* = 100 adults ages ≥65 yr who lived independently and did not use walking or technical aids; *n* = 50 OT training program (*M* age = 81 yr) and usual care (nursing and physical therapy), *n* = 50 control (usual care, no OT; *M* age = 79 yr).	*Intervention* OT provided individualized ADL training for 45–60 min weekday mornings during the hospital stay. A home visit was conducted during inpatient stay (with the participant) to determine how to prepare and adapt the home environment. *Outcome Measures* Klein–Bell ADL scale, Disability Rating Index (ADL/IADL performance).	At 2 mo, all participants regained ADL and IADL abilities. Half of the control group participants received technical aids and home modifications; 90% received preventive changes (e.g., removal of throw rugs.)	Nursing staff was aware of allocation of participants to each group. No information on type of home modifications or how delivered. Individual effect of home modifications in improving functioning is unknown for this multicomponent intervention.
Hendriks et al. (2008)	To determine the effectiveness of a multidisciplinary fall prevention program in preventing falls and functional decline in older adults compared with usual care Pragmatic trial	Level I RCT *N* = 333 older adults ages ≥65 yr who presented to the emergency room after a fall; *n* = 166 intervention (*M* age = 74.5 yr, 66.9% women), *n* = 167 usual care (*M* age = 75.2 yr, 70.1% women).	*Intervention* The intervention included a medical assessment followed by a single in-home functional and environmental assessment by an occupational therapist with written recommendations. Modifications or additional supports were referred to social and community services. Self-reported adherence to referrals and therapist recommendations was 75%. *Outcome Measures* Falls (self-report), Frenchay Activities Index (FAI), Groningen Activity Restriction Scale (GARS), fear of falling, social participation, EuroQual QoL measure.	No statistically significant difference between groups for falls or daily functioning. Daily functioning significantly improved in participants ages ≥80 when comparing intervention group with control group.	No objective observation of function after recommendations; study relied on self-report. Some contamination of the usual care group (MDs treated both groups and may have provided intervention advice to treatment group). Intervention not provided (referral only) and no training provided after recommendations. Potential deviations from protocol. Dropouts (75 participants) were on average older and had lower scores on the FAI.

http://dx.doi.org/10.1111/j.1532-5415.2008.01803.x

(Continued)

Table D1. Home Modification Interventions for Adults and Older Adults (Cont.)

Author/ Year	Study Objectives	Level/Design/ Participants	Intervention and Outcome Measures	Results	Study Limitations
Huang & Acton (2004)	To examine the effect of a multifactorial intervention to prevent falls by increasing self-efficacy to prevent falls, improving the knowledge of medication safety, and decreasing the number of environmental risks in older community-dwelling people	Level I RCT $N = 120$ cognitively intact residents of the community ages ≥65 yr; $n = 60$ intervention (M age = 72.37 yr), $n = 60$ control (M age = 71.58 yr).	*Intervention* Three home visits in a 4-mo period with standardized and individualized fall prevention teaching and an individualized brochure based on fall-related risk factors (medication and environmental safety). *Control*: Standardized fall-prevention brochure. *Outcome Measures* Falls (self-report); falls efficacy (Falls Efficacy Scale); Environmental Hazards checklist (developed for the study).	At 2 mo, the incidence of falls was reduced in both groups, and fall self-efficacy improved for both groups. Fewer self-reported environmental hazards and improved medication knowledge for participants in the treatment group.	The environmental home safety checklist was not a standardized measure. No report of changes made to reduce home hazards during home visits. Outcomes measured only 2 mo after the intervention (typical fall follow-up period is 12 mo). The majority of the participants did not report falls in a 1-yr fall history. No report on who delivered the intervention.

http://dx.doi.org/10.1111/j.0737-1209.2004.21307.x

(Continued)

Table D1. Home Modification Interventions for Adults and Older Adults (*Cont.*)

Author/ Year	Study Objectives	Level/Design/ Participants	Intervention and Outcome Measures	Results	Study Limitations
La Grow, Robertson, Campbell, Clarke, & Kerse (2006)	To examine the efficacy of a home safety program using removal or alteration of hazards and behavioral modification to reduce falls for older adults with severe visual impairment	Level 1 RCT, 2×2 factorial design $N = 391$ people ages ≥ 75 yr with a distance visual acuity of 6/24 m or worse who lived in the community and were ambulatory; $n = 100$ home safety; $n = 97$ Otago exercise program and vitamin D, $n = 98$ exercise and home safety, $n = 96$ social visits.	*Intervention* *Home safety program:* Home safety checklist with discussion on actions for reduction of hazards by an OT. The OT facilitated provision of and payment for new equipment, depending on price and type of item. At follow-up, 90% reported complying partially or completely with 1 or more of the recommendations. *Exercise program:* 1 yr of a modified exercise program with vitamin D supplementation. *Social visits:* 2 hour-long home visits. *Outcome Measures* Falls (hazard and non–hazard related).	Hazard-related and non–hazard-related falls were reduced in the home safety program compared with social visits.	Possible interaction effect between the home safety and exercise programs. No information provided about the number of hazards not resolved.

http://dx.doi.org/10.1136/ip.2006.012252

(Continued)

Table D1. Home Modification Interventions for Adults and Older Adults (*Cont.*)

Author/ Year	Study Objectives	Level/Design/ Participants	Intervention and Outcome Measures	Results	Study Limitations
Lin, Wolf, Hwang, Gong, & Chen (2007)	To compare the effects of 3 fall prevention programs on QoL, functional balance and gait, ADLs, fear of falling, and depression	Level I RCT $N = 150$ adults ages ≥65 yr with a recent fall requiring medical attention in the previous 4 wk (M age = 76.8 yr); $n = 50$ educational group (ED), $n = 50$ home safety assessment and modification group (HSAM; prespecified list of 14 home hazards), $n = 50$ home-based exercise training group (ET).	*Intervention* Interventions were provided in participant's home biweekly for 4 mo. *ED:* Social visit and pamphlets on fall prevention by a public health worker. *HSAM:* Safety assessment and recommendations for home hazard removal by a public health worker. Modifications were provided. *ET:* An individualized stretching, strengthening, and balance training program led by a PT. *Outcome Measures* The Older Americans Resources and Services (OARS) ADL Scale, self-reported falls, World Health Organization Quality of Life instrument (WHOQOL–BREF), fear of falling, Abbreviated Injury Scale (AIS).	The WHOQOL–BREF score changes over the intervention period for the HSAM group improved but were not statistically significant. No difference was found between the HSAM and control groups in risk of falls. The ET group improved significantly for all outcome measures except depression.	It is possible that people improved on scores simply because of physical recovery from their falls rather than because of the intervention provided. Limited follow-up time (4 mo). Results may not generalize to frail older adults because that population tended not to participate or not to remain in the study. Descriptive statistics not available by group. The level of training that public health workers had to identify and resolve home hazards is unknown. Home hazard treatment was not tailored.

http://dx.doi.org/10.1111/j.1532-5415.2007.01146.x

(Continued)

Table D1. Home Modification Interventions for Adults and Older Adults (Cont.)

Author/ Year	Study Objectives	Level/Design/ Participants	Intervention and Outcome Measures	Results	Study Limitations
Mann, Ottenbacher, Fraas, Tomita, & Granger (1999)	To evaluate system of an assistive technology and environmental interventions service provision designed to promote independence and reduce health care costs for physically frail older adults.	Level I RCT $N = 104$ older adults with difficulty in ≥1 area on the FIM Motor scale (M age = 73 yr; 73 women, 31 men); $n = 52$ intervention (M age = 74.3 yr), $n = 52$ control (M age = 71.6 yr).	*Intervention* OTs performed in-home assessments, provided recommendations, and made provisions for the delivery of assistive technologies and environmental modifications. A home modification technician trained participants to safely use the modifications. *Outcome Measures* FIM, Older Americans Research Services Center Instrument, pain as measured using the Functional Status Index (FSI).	At 18 mo, both groups declined in functional status, but the intervention group's decline was significantly less than the control group's decline. Pain increased significantly more in the control group.	Participants in the control group received devices and environmental interventions from other sources. Blinding was difficult to maintain because the research associate was aware of modifications during in-home assessments.

http://dx.doi.org/10.1111/j.1532-5415.2007.01146.x

Author/ Year	Study Objectives	Level/Design/ Participants	Intervention and Outcome Measures	Results	Study Limitations
Nikolaus & Bach (2003)	To assess the effectiveness of a home assessment and intervention program in reducing falls in a community-dwelling, frail, older adult population	Level I RCT $N = 360$ adults admitted from home to a geriatric hospital showing functional decline, especially in mobility (M age = 81.5 yr); $n = 181$ home intervention team (HIT; M age = 81.2 yr), $n = 179$ control (M age = 81.9 yr).	*Intervention* Participants were randomly assigned to a comprehensive geriatric assessment and follow-up home visits or control. *HIT:* Nurse, PT, and OT performed comprehensive geriatric assessment and follow-up home visit. Home hazards identified while the participant was hospitalized and during a follow-up home visit after discharge to remove home hazards and train to safely use environmental modifications (technical and mobility aids); 76% made ≥1 recommended change. *Control:* Comprehensive geriatric assessment with recommendations and usual care at home. *Outcome Measures* Self-reported falls, Barthel Index (ADLs), and Lawton/Brody Questionnaire (IADLs).	The intervention reduced reported falls by 31%. Participants who made ≥1 of the recommended changes experienced a significant reduction in the rate of falls. Sensitivity analysis: the number of falls in intervention group participants with no home modifications was not significantly different from that in the control group. The proportion of frequent fallers (>2 falls) was not significantly different for the intervention and control groups.	Falls were self-reported. Approximately 20% of participants in each group were not followed for the full 12 mo as a result of death, moving to long-term care, or being lost to follow-up.

http://dx.doi.org/10.1046/j.1532-5415.2003.51102.x

(Continued)

Table D1. Home Modification Interventions for Adults and Older Adults (*Cont.*)

Author/ Year	Study Objectives	Level/Design/ Participants	Intervention and Outcome Measures	Results	Study Limitations
Pardessus et al. (2002)	To determine whether home visits by OT reduce the risk of falling and improve the autonomy of older patients hospitalized for falling	Level I RCT $N = 60$ participants who were hospitalized for falling (M age = 83.5 yr); $n = 30$ home intervention (M age = 83.5 yr), $n = 30$ control (M age = 82.9 yr).	*Intervention* A home visit was conducted to identify environmental hazards; modifications recommended. Simple home hazard removal accomplished during assessment if possible. *Outcome Measures* Falls (self-report), hospitalization for falling, institutionalization from fall, and death from fall at 6 and 12 mo; Katz ADL scale; Barberger Gateau et al. IADL scale; functional autonomy measurement system.	The rate of falls, hospitalization for falls, institutionalization, and death were not significantly different between the 2 groups. The decrease in function was significantly more severe in the control group in multiple domains.	Autonomy was defined as independence in ADLs and IADLs. Disagreement with regard to who provided the intervention (stated as OT in abstract, MD in methods). No description of the method of fall ascertainment. No descriptions of the home modification and no report of adherence to home modifications. Sample size not adequate to measure the primary outcome of falls.

http://dx.doi.org/10.1097/00002060-200204000-00002

(Continued)

Table D1. Home Modification Interventions for Adults and Older Adults (*Cont.*)

Author/ Year	Study Objectives	Level/Design/ Participants	Intervention and Outcome Measures	Results	Study Limitations
Petersson, Kottorp, Bergström, & Lilja (2009)	To investigate the longitudinal impact of home modifications on the difficulty of everyday life for people aging with disabilities and whether other factors had an additional impact on difficulty in everyday life for people receiving home modifications	Level II Quasi-experimental pretest–posttest *N* = 103 community-dwelling adults ages ≥40 yr aging with disabilities and in need of home modifications (*M* age = 75.0 yr); *n* = 74 home modifications (*M* age = 75.19 yr, 69% women, 59% lived alone), *n* = 29 control (*M* age = 74.5 yr, 66% women, 66% lived alone).	*Intervention* A wait-list control study of participants in Sweden's Agency for Home Modifications. *Treatment:* OTs interviewed participants before and 2 and 6 mo after receiving home modifications. Areas of intervention included shower, toilet, elevator, ramp, handrail, automatic door openers, and other modifications (unspecified). *Control:* OTs interviewed participants at baseline and repeated the measure at 2 mo and again at 6 mo. *Outcome Measures* Client-Clinical Assessment Protocol Part I (self-rated independence, difficulty, and safety in completing ADLs).	The intervention group experienced less difficulty in everyday life up to 6 mo compared with the comparison group. A small-to-moderate effect size for home modifications was seen in the intervention group. Time waiting for the home modification had an additional impact on experienced difficulties in everyday life.	The sample was limited to those who had already applied for home modifications and may not be generally representative. Psychometric limitations of outcome measure. Potential bias of other interventions or technical assistance available during the study. Difficulty of measuring whether the self-rated improvements in everyday life were a direct consequence of the home modifications.

http://dx.doi.org/10.1080/11038120802409747

(Continued)

Author/Year	Study Objectives	Level/Design/Participants	Intervention and Outcome Measures	Results	Study Limitations
Petersson, Lilja, Hammel, & Kottorp (2008) http://dx.doi.org/10.2340/16501977-0160	To examine the impact of home modifications on self-rated ability in everyday life for people aging with disabilities	Level II Quasi-experimental pretest–posttest *N* = 114 community-dwelling adults ages ≥40 yr in need of home modification for self-care, mobility, or getting in and out of the house (*M* age = 75.3 yr); *n* = 73 home modification program participants (*M* age = 75.7 yr), *n* = 41 wait-list control (*M* age = 74.6 yr).	*Intervention* A wait-list control study of participants in Sweden's Agency for Home Modifications. *Treatment:* OTs interviewed participants before and 2 mo after receiving home modifications. Areas of intervention included shower, toilet, elevator, ramp, handrail, automatic door openers, and other modifications (unspecified). *Control:* OTs interviewed participants at baseline and repeated the measure 2 mo later. *Outcome Measures* Client-Clinical Assessment Protocol Part I (self-rated independence, difficulty, and safety in completing ADLs).	Participants who received home modifications reported a significant improvement in self-rated daily activity abilities and reduced difficulty compared with those in the wait-list group.	The sample was limited to those who had already applied for home modifications and may not be generally representative. Psychometric limitations of outcome measure. Potential bias of other interventions or technical assistance available during the study. Difficulty in measuring whether the self-rated improvements in everyday life were a direct consequence of the home modifications.
Pighills, Torgerson, Sheldon, Drummond, & Bland (2011) http://dx.doi.org/10.1111/j.1532-5415.2010.03221.x	To compare the efficacy of an environmental falls prevention intervention delivered by OTs and trained assessors	Level I Pilot 3-armed RCT *N* = 238 community-dwelling adults ages ≥70 yr with a history of ≥1 falls in the previous year; *n* = 73 trained assessor–conducted (e.g., nurses aid) home hazard assessment (*M* age = 79 yr), *n* = 87 OT–conducted home hazard assessment (*M* age = 78 yr), *n* = 78 control (*M* age = 80 yr).	*Intervention* The Westmead Home Safety Assessment (WeHSA) was conducted in the participant's home. Potential falls hazards were discussed and minor hazards resolved during the visit. A written report was provided to the participant, and referrals were made for removing hazards. A significantly greater number of recommendations were made and adhered to in the OT group. *Outcome Measures* Fall (self-report); fear of falling; Barthel Index.	Fall rate in the OT group was approximately half that of the controls, but the trained assessor group was not significantly different from the control group. No difference was found in independence in ADLs between the trained assessor or OT group and controls.	Cognition was not assessed in the sample.

(Continued)

Table D1. Home Modification Interventions for Adults and Older Adults (*Cont.*)

Author/ Year	Study Objectives	Level/Design/ Participants	Intervention and Outcome Measures	Results	Study Limitations
Plautz, Beck, Selmar, & Radetsky (1996)	To determine whether minor home safety modifications decreased rates of falls, scalds, and burns	Level III Single-group pretest–posttest $N = 141$ people ages ≥75 yr with 0–6 falls or ages ≥60 yr with 1–6 falls in the past year (M age = 75.3 years, 84% women).	*Intervention* Fall and injury rates were prospectively collected on a calendar for 6 mo; participants received treatment, and fall and injury rates were collected for an additional 6 mo. Participants received counseling and written material on injury risk factors from a VISTA outreach worker. Homes were assessed using a detailed safety assessment checklist. The interventionists made recommendations and assisted clients in some interventions. *Outcome Measures* Self-report of falls, burns, and scalds.	The rate of falls was reduced 59% in the follow-up period. Scalds and burns were decreased significantly. The rate of combined falls, burns, and scalds was significantly reduced.	Incomplete data for many participants. No detailed information on the falls that were reported and likely that falls were underreported. No information on the qualifications of the outreach worker performing intervention.
Poulstrup & Jeune (2000)	To determine the effectiveness of a community-based intervention program to reduce the number of fall injuries requiring hospital treatment	Level II Nonrandomized pretest–posttest Community-dwelling older adults ages ≥65 yr; $n = 12,905$ intervention group, $n = 11,460$ control group.	*Intervention* Multicomponent intervention including written and verbal fall prevention information on fall risk factors (physical hazards, somatic illness and age debilities, psychiatric illness, drug consumption, diet insufficiency, and inactivity) was delivered to all older adults in treatment community. Home visits by nurses, general practitioners, and home helpers were provided to identify and educate on home hazards for 70- to 79-year-old participants or those using home help.	46% reduction in fracture for women in the treatment group compared with the control group. No difference in fractures in men in treatment group compared with the control group.	No details on the home hazard removal program or the intervention or adherence rates of the program. No information provided on the qualifications of the home helpers. It is estimated information on fall prevention only reached 60%–70% of the population. Effect of home modification difficult to ascertain because only 25% of the population received changes to physical surroundings or medication changes and disease treatment.

http://dx.doi.org/10.1093/eurpub/10.1.45

(Continued)

Table D1. Home Modification Interventions for Adults and Older Adults (*Cont.*)

Author/ Year	Study Objectives	Level/Design/ Participants	Intervention and Outcome Measures	Results	Study Limitations
Stark (2004)	To examine the effect of a home modification program that included architectural modification and adaptive equipment for community-dwelling older adults with disabilities	Level III Nonrandomized pretest–posttest design *N* = 29 low-income older adults with functional limitations (*M* age = 67.3 yr.	*Intervention* Participants received a comprehensive assessment of abilities and environmental barriers. A tailored treatment plan was developed in collaboration with the participant. The modifications were provided with the therapist training participants in modification use. *Outcome Measures* FIM, COPM, Environmental Functional Independence Measure (EFIM).	Participants' occupational performance scores went up significantly postintervention. Scores on satisfaction with performance increased significantly.	Small sample size. The sample is not representative of the general population. Some large time lapses between initial evaluation and provision of home modifications may have allowed changes in physical status to affect results. Only 60% of the recommendations on barrier removal were completed.
Stark, Landsbaum, Palmer, Somerville, & Morris (2009)	To describe a client-centered OT home modification intervention program and examine the impact on functional performance over time	Level III Quasi-experimental design, pretest–posttest–posttest prospective study *N* = 67 participants ages ≥60 yr and older with functional limitations (*M* age = 81.7 yr, 88% women).	*Intervention* OT completed a structured in-home evaluation. Home modifications, assistive technology, education, and follow-up training were provided. 80% of recommendations were followed. *Outcome Measures* FIM.	A significant increase in functional independence, performance, and satisfaction with performance at 1 mo. No change in functional independence and performance from posttest to 2-yr follow-up.	Small sample size, no control group. Treating therapist as single unblinded rater. Inability to control other supportive changes. Fairly healthy, community-dwelling, White population.

(Continued)

Table D1. Home Modification Interventions for Adults and Older Adults (*Cont.*)

Author/ Year	Study Objectives	Level/Design/ Participants	Intervention and Outcome Measures	Results	Study Limitations
Tinetti et al. (1999)	To determine whether a home-based systematic multicomponent rehabilitation strategy leads to improved outcomes relative to usual care	Level I RCT $N = 304$ people without dementia ages ≥65 yr who underwent surgical repair of a hip fracture and returned home within 100 days; $n = 148$ systematic multicomponent rehabilitation by physical therapist and nursing (M age = 80.5 yr), $n = 156$ usual care (M age = 79.4).	*Intervention* Intervention group received home-based therapy including PT for strengthening and functional therapy by a nurse (based on OT principles) that included task modification, use of adaptive equipment, environmental modifications, psychological interventions (to enhance confidence or motivation), caregiver (usually family) education and involvement, and referral. *Usual care:* Traditional home health services. *Outcome Measures* Occupational Therapy Functional Assessment Compilation (OTFACT), self-reported falls.	No significant difference was found between groups in ADL performance.	Daily activity task analysis and treatment provided by nurse in the treatment group. No description of the intervention, home assessment process, type of modifications, or adherence to modifications provided.
Tomita, Mann, Stanton, Tomita, & Sundar (2007) http://dx.doi.org/10.1016/S0003-9993(99)90083-7	To determine whether residents of smart homes (SHs) maintain physical and cognitive functions better than non-SH residents and whether the rate of living independently at home is higher for SH residents	Level I RCT $N = 78$ adults ages ≥60 yr living alone with difficulty in ADLs or IADLs and interest in using a computer; $n = 34$ treatment group (M age = 72 yr, 88.2% women, 70.6% White), $n = 44$ control (M age = 75.6 yr, 88% women, 81.8% White).	*Intervention* A 2.5-hr home assessment was completed by an OT or a nurse. The home was retrofitted with door and window sensors, a motion sensor, a power flash for the security system and alarm (chime), and a wall switch for manual control for lighting connected to a motion detector. Support to use the device was provided. *Outcome Measures* FIM, OARS IADL Scale, mobility subsection of dysfunction section of Sickness Impact Profile (SIP), Craig Handicap Assessment and Reporting Technique (CHART) mobility for handicap measure, Mini-Mental State Examination (MMSE).	The treatment group was significantly younger than the control group, and the control group had a higher rate of comorbid conditions. No visits provided to the control group. Use of OT or nurse for home assessment. High attrition rate (treatment group, 26%; control group, 34%).	Intervention and control groups received additional in-home services (nursing and rehabilitation). No report of comparison of those who dropped out to those who remained in the study.

(Continued)

Table D1. Home Modification Interventions for Adults and Older Adults *(Cont.)*

Author/ Year	Study Objectives	Level/Design/ Participants	Intervention and Outcome Measures	Results	Study Limitations
van Haastregt et al. (2000)	To evaluate whether a program of multifactorial home visits reduces falls and impairments in mobility in older adults living in the community	Level I RCT $N = 316$ people ages ≥70 yr living in the community with moderate mobility impairments or history of ≥2 falls in the previous 6 mo; $n = 159$ intervention group (M age = 77.2 yr, 62% with below-average income), $n = 157$ control group (M age = 77.2 yr, 66% with below-average income).	*Intervention* Five home visits over 1 yr completed by nurses to screen for medical, environmental, and behavioral factors. Participants were given advice and referrals to resolve hazards. Follow-ups were at 12 and 18 months. In comparison, the usual-care group did not experience any fall prevention efforts. *Outcome Measures* Falls (self-report), Mobility Control scale and Mobility Range scale of the SIP, FAI, Falls Efficacy Scale.	No difference was found in fall risk between the groups. The intervention group showed significantly less decline in daily activity than those in the control group at 12 mo. At 18 mo, this effect was no longer significant. The intervention group had significantly less fear of falling than the control group.	Lack of adherence by intervention group participants. Dropouts during the follow-up period included those anticipated to benefit most from the intervention. Increase in risk behavior may have influenced results because the intervention group had less fear of falling and more activity level than control group. Lack of inclusion of enough extra elements outside of usual care.

http://dx.doi.org/10.1136/bmj.321.7267.994

(Continued)

Table D1. Home Modification Interventions for Adults and Older Adults *(Cont.)*

Author/ Year	Study Objectives	Level/Design/ Participants	Intervention and Outcome Measures	Results	Study Limitations
Velligan et al. (2008)	To compare the efficacy of providing CAT and GES to standard treatment for community-dwelling people with schizophrenia and to determine whether improvements are maintained with reduction in frequency in CAT	Level I RCT N = 120 people with a diagnosis of schizophrenia or schizoaffective disorder, use of an atypical antipsychotic medication other than clozapine, no hospitalizations, and a stable living environment for the past 3 mo (ages 18–60, M age = 41 yr), n = 40 CAT (M age = 41 yr), n = 40 GES (M age = 42 yr), n = 40 treatment as usual (M age = 40 yr).	*Intervention* *CAT:* Customized compensatory strategies based on comprehensive assessment and weekly home visits (30 min) and environmental supports provided at home over 9 mo. *GES:* Manual-driven series of environmental supports provided in a clinic. *TAU:* Treatment-as-usual control group. Intervention delivered by an OT. *Outcome Measures* Social and Occupational Functioning Scale (SOFS), Multnomah Community Ability Scale (MCAS).	The CAT group demonstrated a large effect size and the GES group demonstrated a medium effect size compared with the TAU group. Treatment gains decreased with reduction of session frequency.	Length of illness for participants (average time was more than a decade). Rating of symptoms irrespective of origin.
Velligan et al. (2009)	To examine the short-term efficacy of CAT, GES, and treatment as usual	Level I RCT N = 120 adults ages 18–60 yr with schizophrenia or schizoaffective disorder receiving services from community clinics; n = 39 usual-treatment group (M age 40 yr), n = 38 GES (M age = 42), n = 36 CAT (M age = 41).	*Intervention* *CAT:* Manual-driven series of environmental supports based on a comprehensive assessment of abilities and environment. *GES:* A generic set of environmental supports. *TAU:* Treatment-as-usual control group. *Outcome Measures* Adherence and utilization (monthly phone contact), SOFS, MCAS.	CAT group differed significantly from the TAU group and had an improved mean SOFAS at 3 mo. GES group differed significantly from TAU group and had improved SOFAS at 3 mo. CAT participants used a higher proportion of supports than GES participants. CAT participants were more likely to improve specific target behaviors than GES participants. Participants in both groups who had higher utilization rates had improved scores on SOFAS.	Researchers were aware of treatment group assignment. Study relied on self-report to assess medication adherence. The length of follow-up was 3 mo.

http://dx.doi.org/10.1016/j.psychres.2008.03.016

(Continued)

Table D1. Home Modification Interventions for Adults and Older Adults (*Cont.*)

Author/ Year	Study Objectives	Level/Design/ Participants	Intervention and Outcome Measures	Results	Study Limitations
Wilson, Mitchell, Kemp, Adkins, & Mann (2009) http://dx.doi.org/10.1080/10400430903246068	To determine the effect of an assistive technology program on function and rate of decline for people with early-onset disability	Level I RCT *N* = 91 people who reported a need for equipment; had major muscle weakness, mobility problems, upper-extremity pain; or reported pain or fatigue that interfered with function (68 women, 23 men, *M* age = 62 yr, age range = 30–89 yr); *n* = 47 intervention (*M* age = 62), *n* = 44 control (*M* age = 62). Impairments included polio, spinal cord injury, rheumatoid arthritis, and other (cerebral palsy, stroke, and peripheral neuropathy).	*Intervention* In-home assessment by an OT and equipment specialist with recommendations for specific home modifications, assistive technology, or behavior modifications. For the majority, devices and necessary training were provided. New assistive technology and assistance were available throughout the study. *Outcome Measures* OARS, FIM.	A significant increase in caregiver hours occurred over time for both groups. Both groups showed functional decline with significant time findings for FIM and IADL scores over time. The treatment group showed a slower decline in function and reported significantly more desired functional changes at 12 mo.	Small sample size may prevent generalizability. The use of adaptive equipment (the intervention) is penalized by the primary outcome measures and thus may artificially reduce the outcome of the intervention. Control group able to independently obtain assistive technology. Delay in delivery of environmental modification and assistive technology. Blinding of interviews over the entire study not viable.

Note. AD = Alzheimer's disease; ADL/ADLs = activity/activities of daily living; CAT = cognitive adaptive training; GES = generic environmental supports; IADL/IADLs = instrumental activity/activities of daily living; *M* = mean; MD = physician; mo = month/months; OT = occupational therapy/therapist; PT = physical therapy/therapist; QoL = quality of life; RCT = randomized controlled trial; yr = year/years.

References

Accreditation Council for Occupational Therapy Education. (2012). 2011 Accreditation Council for Occupational Therapy Education (ACOTE®) standards. *American Journal of Occupational Therapy, 66*(6, Suppl.), S6–S74. http://dx.doi/org/10.5014/ajot.2013.67S9

Agency for Healthcare Research and Quality, U.S. Preventive Task Force. (2012). *Grade definitions.* Retrieved from http://www.uspreventive servicestaskforce.org/uspstf/grades.htm

Alexander, B. H., Rivara, F. P., & Wolf, M. E. (1992). The cost and frequency of hospitalization for fall-related injuries in older adults. *American Journal of Public Health, 82,* 1020–1023. http://dx.doi.org/10.2105/AJPH.82.7.1020

American Medical Association. (2013). *CPT 2014.* Chicago: Author.

American Occupational Therapy Association. (1989). Uniform terminology for occupational therapy (2nd ed.). *American Journal of Occupational Therapy, 43,* 808–815. http://dx.doi.org/10.5014/ajot.43.12.808

American Occupational Therapy Association. (1994). Uniform terminology for occupational therapy (3rd ed.). *American Journal of Occupational Therapy, 48,* 1047–1054. http://dx.doi.org/10.5014/ajot.48.11.1047

American Occupational Therapy Association. (2002). Occupational therapy practice framework: Domain and process. *American Journal of Occupational Therapy, 56,* 609–639. http://dx.doi.org/10.5014/ajot.56.6.609

American Occupational Therapy Association. (2006). Policy 1.44: Categories of occupational therapy personnel. In *Policy manual* (2013 ed., pp. 32–33). Bethesda, MD: Author.

American Occupational Therapy Association. (2008). Occupational therapy practice framework: Domain and process (2nd ed.). *American Journal of Occupational Therapy, 62,* 625–683. http://dx.doi.org/10.5014/ajot.62.6.625

American Occupational Therapy Association. (2009). Guidelines for supervision, roles, and responsibilities during the delivery of therapy services. *American Journal of Occupational Therapy, 58,* 663–667. http://dx.doi.org/10.5014/ajot.63.6.797

American Occupational Therapy Association. (2010). Standards of practice for occupational therapy. *American Journal of Occupational Therapy, 64*(Suppl.), S106–S111. http://dx.doi.org/10.5014/ajot.2010.64S106

American Occupational Therapy Association. (2013a). Cognition, cognitive rehabilitation, and occupational performance. *American Journal of Occupational Therapy, 67*(Suppl.), S9–S31. http://dx.doi.org/10.5014/ajot.2013.67S9

American Occupational Therapy Association. (2013b). Guidelines for documentation of occupational therapy. *American Journal of Occupational Therapy, 67*(Suppl.), S32–S38. http://dx.doi.org/10.5014/ajot.2013.67S32

American Occupational Therapy Association. (2014). Occupational therapy practice framework: Domain and process (3rd ed.). *American Journal of Occupational Therapy, 68*(Suppl. 1), S1–S48. http://dx.doi.org/10.5014/ajot.2014.682006

Americans With Disabilities Act of 1990, Pub. L. 101–336, 42 U.S.C. § 12101.

Arfken, C. L., Lach, H. W., Birge, S. J., & Miller, J. P. (1994). The prevalence and correlates of fear of falling in elderly persons living in the community. *American Journal of Public Health, 84,* 565–570. http://dx.doi.org/10.2105/AJPH.84.4.565

Baum, C., & Edwards, D. (2008). *Activity Card Sort* (2nd ed.). Bethesda, MD: AOTA Press.

Blumenthal, B. (2003). *Investing in capacity building: A guide to high-impact approaches.* New York: Foundation Center.

Brotman, D. J., Golden, S. H., & Wittstein, I. S. (2007). The cardiovascular toll of stress. *Lancet, 370,* 1089–1100. http://dx.doi.org/10.1016/S0140-6736(07)61305-1

Brunnström, G., Sörensen, S., Alsterstad, K., & Sjöstrand, J. (2004). Quality of light and quality of life—The effect of lighting adaptation among people with low vision. *Ophthalmic and Physiological Optics, 24,* 274–280. http://dx.doi.org/10.1111/j.1475-1313.2004.00192.x

Campbell, A. J., Robertson, M. C., La Grow, S. J., Kerse, N. M., Sanderson, G. F., Jacobs, R. J., . . . Hale, L. A. (2005). Randomised controlled trial of prevention of falls in people aged > or =75 with severe visual impairment: The VIP trial. *BMJ, 331,* 817. http://dx.doi.org/10.1136/bmj.38601.447731.55

Charlson, M. E., Pompei, P., Ales, K. L., & MacKenzie, C. R. (1987). A new method of classifying prognostic comorbidity in longitudinal studies: Development and validation. *Journal of Chronic Diseases, 40,* 373–383. http://dx.doi.org/10.1016/0021-9681(87)90171-8

Chiu, T., Oliver, R., Ascott, P., Choo, L. C., Davis, T., Gaya, A., . . . Letts, L. (2006). *Safety Assessment of Function and the Environment for Rehabilitation (SAFER) Health Outcome Measurement and Evaluation (HOME), version 3.* Toronto: COTA Health.

Christenson, M. (1991). Lifease [Computer software]. Minneapolis: Lifease.

Christenson, M. (2006). Buildease [Computer software]. Minneapolis: Lifease.

Clemson, L. (1997). *Home fall hazards and the Westmead Home Safety Assessment (WESHA).* West Brunswick, Australia: Coordinates Publications.

Clemson, L., Cumming, R. G., Kendig, H., Swann, M., Heard, R., & Taylor, K. (2004). The effectiveness of a community-based program for reducing the incidence of falls in the elderly: A randomized trial. *Journal of the American Geriatrics Society, 52,* 1487–1494. http://dx.doi.org/10.1111/j.1532-5415.2004.52411.x

Clemson, L., Mackenzie, L., Ballinger, C., Close, J. C., & Cumming, R. G. (2008). Environmental interventions to prevent falls in community-dwelling older people: A meta-analysis of randomized trials. *Journal of Aging and Health, 20,* 954–971. http://dx.doi.org/10.1177/0898264308324672

Clemson, L., Singh, M. A. F., Bundy, A., Cumming, R. G., Manollaras, K., Loughlin, P., & Black, D. (2012). Integration of balance and strength training into daily life activity to reduce rate of falls in older people (the LiFE study): Randomised parallel trial. *BMJ, 345,* e4547. http://dx.doi.org/10.1136bmj.e4547

Close, J., Ellis, M., Hooper, R., Glucksman, E., Jackson, S., & Swift, C. (1999). Prevention of Falls in the Elderly Trial (PROFET): A randomised controlled trial. *Lancet, 353,* 93–97.

Connell, B. R., & Sanford, J. (1997). Individualizing home modification recommendations to facilitate performance of routine activities. In S. Laspry & J. Hyde (Eds.), *Staying put, adapting the places to the people* (pp. 113–131). Amityville, NY: Baywood.

Cooper Marcus, C. (1997). *House as a mirror of self: Exploring the deeper meaning of home*. Berkeley, CA: Conari Press.

Costa, P. T., & McCrae, R. R. (1992). *Revised NEO Personality Inventory (NEO PI–R) and NEO Five-Factor Inventory (NEO–FFI)*. Odessa, FL: Psychological Assessment Resources.

Cumming, R. G., Thomas, M., Szonyi, G., Salkeld, G., O'Neill, E., Westbury, C., & Frampton, G. (1999). Home visits by an occupational therapist for assessment and modification of environmental hazards: A randomized trial of falls prevention. *Journal of the American Geriatrics Society, 47*, 1397–1402.

Davison, J., Bond, J., Dawson, P., Steen, I. N., & Kenny, R. A. (2005). Patients with recurrent falls attending Accident and Emergency benefit from multifactorial intervention: A randomised controlled trial. *Age and Ageing, 34*, 162–168. http://dx.doi.org/10.1093/ageing/afi053

Donelan, K., Hill, C. A., Hoffman, C., Scoles, K., Feldman, P. H., Levine, C., & Gould, D. (2002). Challenged to care: Informal caregivers in a changing health system. *Health Affairs, 21*, 222–231. http://dx.doi.org/10.1377/hlthaff.21.4.222

Dooley, N. R., & Hinojosa, J. (2004). Improving quality of life for persons with Alzheimer's disease and their family caregivers: Brief occupational therapy intervention. *American Journal of Occupational Therapy, 58*, 561–569. http://dx.doi.org/10.5014/ajot.58.5.561

Dovey, K. (1985). Home and homelessness. In I. Altman & C. Werner (Eds.), *Home environments: Human behavior and environment advances in theory and research* (Vol. 8, pp. 33–64). New York: Springer.

Dunn, W., McClain, L. H., Brown, C., & Youngstrom, M. J. (1998). The ecology of human performance. In M. E. Neistadt & E. B. Crepeau (Eds.), *Willard and Spackman's occupational therapy* (9th ed., pp. 525–535). Philadelphia: Lippincott Williams & Wilkins.

Fair Housing Act Amendments of 1988, Pub. L. No. 100–430, 102 Stat. 1619.

Fänge, A., & Iwarsson, S. (2005). Changes in ADL dependence and aspects of usability following housing adaptation: A longitudinal perspective. *American Journal of Occupational Therapy, 59*, 296–304. http://dx.doi.org/10.5014/ajot.59.3.296

Federal Interagency Forum on Aging-Related Statistics. (2012). *Older Americans 2012: Key indicators of well-being*. Washington, DC: U.S. Government Printing Office. Retrieved from http://www.agingstats.gov/agingstatsdotnet/main_site/default.aspx

Fiese, B. H. (2007). Routines and rituals: Opportunities for participation in family health. *OTJR: Occupation, Participation and Health, 27*, S41–S49.

Fiese, B. H., Tomcho, T. J., Douglas, M., Josephs, K., Poltrock, S., & Baker, T. (2002). A review of 50 years of research on naturally occurring family routines and rituals: Cause for celebration? *Journal of Family Psychology, 16*, 381–390.

Fisher, A. (1995). *Assessment of Motor and Process Skills*. Fort Collins, CO: Three Star Press.

Fisher, A. G., & Griswold, L. A. (2014). Performance skills: Implementing performance analyses to evaluate quality of occupational performance. In B. A. Boyt Schell, G. Gillen, & M. Scaffa (Eds.), *Willard and Spackman's occupational therapy* (12th ed., pp. 249–264). Philadelphia: Lippincott Williams & Wilkins.

Gillespie, L. D., Robertson, M. C., Gillespie, W. J., Sherrington, C., Gates, S., Clemson, L. M., & Lamb, S. E. (2012). Interventions for preventing falls in older people living in the community. *Cochrane Database of Systematic Reviews, 9*, CD007146.

Gitlin, L. N., Corcoran, M., Winter, L., Boyce, A., & Hauck, W. W. (2001). A randomized, controlled trial of a home environmental intervention: Effect on efficacy and upset in caregivers and on daily function of persons with dementia. *Gerontologist, 41,* 4–14. http://dx.doi.org/10.1093/geront/41.1.4

Gitlin, L. N., Miller, K. S., & Boyce, A. (1999). Bathroom modifications for frail elderly renters: Outcomes of a community-based program. *Technology and Disability, 10,* 141–149.

Gitlin, L., Schinfeld, S., Winter, L., Corcoran, M., Boyce, A., & Hauck, W. (2002). Evaluating home environments of persons with dementia: Interrater reliability and validity of the Home Environment Assessment Protocol (HEAP). *Disability and Rehabilitation, 24,* 59–71.

Gitlin, L. N., Winter, L., Corcoran, M., Dennis, M. P., Schinfeld, S., & Hauck, W. W. (2003). Effects of the Home Environmental Skill-Building Program on the caregiver–care recipient dyad: 6-month outcomes from the Philadelphia REACH Initiative. *Gerontologist, 43,* 532–546. http://dx.doi.org/10.1093/geront/43.4.532

Gitlin, L. N., Winter, L., Dennis, M. P., Corcoran, M., Schinfeld, S., & Hauck, W. W. (2006). A randomized trial of a multicomponent home intervention to reduce functional difficulties in older adults. *Journal of the American Geriatrics Society, 54,* 809–816. http://dx.doi.org/10.1111/j.1532-5415.2006.00703.x

Goffman, E. (1959). *The presentation of self in everyday life.* New York: Doubleday.

Graff, M. J. L., Vernooij-Dassen, M. J. M., Hoefnagels, W. H. L., Dekker, J., & de Witte, L. P. (2003). Occupational therapy at home for older individuals with mild to moderate cognitive impairments and their primary caregivers: A pilot study. *OTJR: Occupation, Participation and Health, 23,* 155–164.

Graff, M. J. L., Vernooij-Dassen, M. J. M, Thijssen, M., Dekker, J., Hoefnagels, W. H., & Rikkert, M. G. (2006). Community-based occupational therapy for patients with dementia and their care givers: Randomised controlled trial. *BMJ, 333,* 1196. http://dx.doi.org/10.1136/bmj.39001.688843.BE

Hagsten, B., Svensson, O., & Gardulf, A. (2004). Early individualized postoperative occupational therapy training in 100 patients improves ADL after hip fracture: A randomized trial. *Acta Orthopaedica Scandinavica, 75,* 177–183.

Harrison-Felix, C. (2001). *The Craig Hospital Inventory of Environmental Factors.* San Jose, CA: Center for Outcome Measurement in Brain Injury.

Hasselkus, B. (2011). *Meaning of everyday occupation* (2nd ed.). Thorofare, NJ: Slack.

Hendriks, M. R., Bleijlevens, M. H., van Haastregt, J. C., Crebolder, H. F., Diederiks, J. P., Evers, S. M., . . . van Eijk, J. T. (2008). Lack of effectiveness of a multidisciplinary fall-prevention program in elderly people at risk: A randomized, controlled trial. *Journal of the American Geriatrics Society, 56,* 1390–1397. http://dx.doi.org/10.1111/j.1532-5415.2008.01803.x

Hislop, H., & Montgomery, J. (2007). *Muscle testing: Techniques of manual examination* (8th ed.). Philadelphia: W. B. Saunders.

Hoenig, H., Sanford, J. A., Butterfield, T., Griffiths, P. C., Richardson, P., & Hargraves, K. (2006). Development of a teletechnology protocol for in-home rehabilitation. *Journal of Rehabilitation Research and Development, 43,* 287–298. http://dx.doi.org/10.1682/JRRD.2004.07.0089

Huang, T. T., & Acton, G. J. (2004). Effectiveness of home visit falls prevention strategy for Taiwanese community-dwelling elders: Randomized trial. *Public Health Nursing, 21,* 247–256. http://dx.doi.org/10.1111/j.0737-1209.2004.21307.x

Iwarsson, S., & Slaug, B. (2001). *The Housing Enabler: An instrument for assessing and analysing accessibility problems in housing.* Nävlinge och Staffanstorp, Sweden: Veten & Stapen HB & Slaug Data Management.

Iwarsson, S., & Stähl, A. (2003). Accessibility, usability and universal design-Positioning and definition of concepts describing person–environment relationships. *Disability and Rehabilitation, 25,* 57–66.

Katzman, R., Brown, T., Fuld, P., Peck, A., Schechter, R., & Schimmel, H. (1983). Validation of a short orientation memory concentration test of cognitive impairment. *American Journal of Psychiatry, 140,* 734–739.

Kraskowsky, L. H., & Finlayson, M. (2001). Factors affecting older adults' use of adaptive equipment: Review of the literature. *American Journal of Occupational Therapy, 55,* 303–310. http://dx.doi.org/10.5014/ajot.55.3.303

Krieger, J., & Higgins, D. L. (2002). Housing and health: Time again for public health action. *American Journal of Public Health, 92,* 758–768. http://dx.doi.org/10.2105/AJPH.92.5.758

La Grow, S. J., Robertson, M. C., Campbell, A. J., Clarke, G. A., & Kerse, N. M. (2006). Reducing hazard related falls in people 75 years and older with significant visual impairment: How did a successful program work? *Injury Prevention, 12,* 296–301. http://dx.doi.org/10.1136/ip.2006.012252

LaPlante, M. P., Harrington, C., & Kang, T. (2002). Estimating paid and unpaid hours of personal assistance services in activities of daily living provided to adults living at home. *Health Services Research, 37,* 397–415.

LaPlante, M. P., Kaye, H. S., Kang, T., & Harrington, C. (2004). Unmet need for personal assistance services: Estimating the shortfall in hours of help and adverse consequences. *Journals of Gerontology, Series B: Psychological Sciences and Social Sciences, 59,* S98–S108. http://dx.doi.org/10.1093/geronb/59.2.S98

Law, M., Baptiste, S., Carswell, A., McColl, M., Polatajko, H., & Pollock, N. (2005). *Canadian Occupational Performance Measure* (4th ed.). Ottawa: CAOT Publications.

Lawton, M. P., & Nahemow, L. (1973). Ecology and the aging process. In C. Eisdorfer & M. P. Lawton (Eds.), *Psychology of adult development and aging* (pp. 619–674). Washington, DC: American Psychological Association.

Lieberman, D., & Scheer, J. (2002). AOTA's Evidence-Based Literature Review Project: An overview. *American Journal of Occupational Therapy, 56,* 344–349. http://dx.doi.org/10.5014/ajot.56.3.344

Lin, M. R., Wolf, S. L., Hwang, H. F., Gong, S. Y., & Chen, C. Y. (2007). A randomized, controlled trial of fall prevention programs and quality of life in older fallers. *Journal of the American Geriatrics Society, 55,* 499–506. http://dx.doi.org/10.1111/j.1532-5415.2007.01146.x

MacKenzie, L., Byles, J., & Higginbotham, N. (2000). Designing the Home Falls and Accidents Screening Tool (HOMEFAST): Selecting the items. *British Journal of Occupational Therapy, 63,* 260–269.

Mann, W. C., Hurren, D., Tomita, M., Bengali, M., & Steinfeld, E. (1994). Environmental problems in homes of elders with disabilities. *OTJR: Occupation, Participation and Health, 14,* 191–211.

Mann, W. C., Ottenbacher, K. J., Fraas, L., Tomita, M., & Granger, C. V. (1999). Effectiveness of assistive technology and environmental interventions in maintaining independence and reducing home care costs for the frail elderly: A randomized controlled trial. *Archives of Family*

Medicine, 8, 210–217. http://dx.doi.org/10.1001/archfami.8.3.210

Mathias, S., Nayak, U. S., & Isaacs, B. (1986). Balance in elderly patients: The "Get-Up and Go" test. *Archives of Physical Medicine and Rehabilitation, 67,* 387–389.

Minkel, J. L. (1996). Assistive technology and outcome measurement: Where do we begin? *Technology and Disability, 5,* 285–288.

Moyers, P., & Dale, L. (2007). *The guide to occupational therapy practice* (2nd ed.). Bethesda, MD: AOTA Press.

Nicol, S., Roys, M., Davidson, M., Summers, C., Ormandy, D., & Ambrose, P. (2010). *Quantifying the cost of poor housing.* Watford, England: IHS BRE Press.

Nikolaus, T., & Bach, M. (2003). Preventing falls in community-dwelling frail older people using a home intervention team (HIT): Results from the randomized Falls–HIT trial. *Journal of the American Geriatrics Society, 51,* 300–305. http://dx.doi.org/10.1046/j.1532-5415.2003.51102.x

Pardessus, V., Puisieux, F., Di Pompeo, C., Gaudefroy, C., Thevenon, A., & Dewailly, P. (2002). Benefits of home visits for falls and autonomy in the elderly: A randomized trial study. *American Journal of Physical Medicine and Rehabilitation, 81,* 247–252. http://dx.doi.org/10.1097/00002060-200204000-00002

Petersson, I., Kottorp, A., Bergström, J., & Lilja, M. (2009). Longitudinal changes in everyday life after home modifications for people aging with disabilities. *Scandinavian Journal of Occupational Therapy, 16,* 78–87. http://dx.doi.org/10.1080/11038120802409747

Petersson, I., Lilja, M., Hammel, J., & Kottorp, A. (2008). Impact of home modification services on ability in everyday life for people ageing with disabilities. *Journal of Rehabilitation Medicine, 40,* 253–260.

Pighills, A. C., Torgerson, D. J., Sheldon, T. A., Drummond, A. E., & Bland, J. M. (2011). Environmental assessment and modification to prevent falls in older people. *Journal of the American Geriatrics Society, 59,* 26–33. http://dx.doi.org/10.1111/j.1532-5415.2010.03221.x

Plautz, B., Beck, D. E., Selmar, C., & Radetsky, M. (1996). Modifying the environment: A community-based injury-reduction program for elderly residents. *American Journal of Preventive Medicine, 12*(Suppl.), 33–38.

Poulstrup, A., & Jeune, B. (2000). Prevention of fall injuries requiring hospital treatment among community-dwelling elderly. *European Journal of Public Health, 10,* 45–50. http://dx.doi.org/10.1093/eurpub/10.1.45

Prochaska, J. O., & Velicer, W. F. (1997). The transtheoretical model of health behavior change. *American Journal of Health Promotion, 12,* 38–48. http://dx.doi.org/10.4278/0890-1171-12.1.38

Radomski, M. V. (1995). There is more to life than putting on your pants. *American Journal of Occupational Therapy, 49,* 487–490. http://dx.doi.org/10.5014/ajot.49.6.487

Rebuilding Together. (n.d.-a). *Our history.* Retrieved from http://rebuildingtogether.org/whoweare/history/

Rebuilding Together. (n.d.-b). *Our mission and vision.* Retrieved from http://rebuildingtogether.org/whoweare/our-mission-and-vision/

Rogers, J., & Holm, M. (1994). *The Performance Assessment of Self-Care Skills (PASS), version 3.1.* Pittsburgh: University of Pittsburgh.

Rogers, J. C., Holm, M. B., Raina, K. D., Dew, M. A., Shih, M.-M., Begley, A., . . . Reynolds, C. F., III. (2010). Disability in late-life major depression: Patterns of self-reported task abilities, task habits, and observed task performance. *Psy-*

chiatry Research, 178, 475–479. http://dx.doi. org/10.1016/j.psychres.2009.11.002

Rowles, G. D. (1991). Beyond performance: Being in place as a component of occupational therapy. *American Journal of Occupational Therapy, 45*, 265–271. http://dx.doi.org/10.5014/ajot.45.3.265

Rowles, G. D. (2000). Habituation and being in place. *OTJR: Occupation, Participation and Health, 20*(Suppl.), S52–S67.

Rowles, G. D. (2008). Place in occupational science: A life course perspective on the role of environmental context in the quest for meaning. *Journal of Occupational Science, 15*, 127–135. http://dx.doi.org/10.1080/14427591.2008.96866 22

Sackett, D. L., Rosenberg, W. M., Muir Gray, J. A., Haynes, R. B., & Richardson, W. S. (1996). Evidence-based medicine: What it is and what it isn't. *BMJ, 312*, 71–72. http://dx.doi.org/10.1136/bmj.312.7023.71

Sanford, J. A., Pynoos, J., Tejral, A., & Browne, A. (2001). Development of a comprehensive assessment for delivery of home modifications. *Physical and Occupational Therapy in Geriatrics, 20*, 43–54. http://dx.doi.org/10.1080/J148v20n02_03

Schawe, K. M., & Crist, P. A. (2013, April). *Home modification practice: A survey of current topics and trends*. Paper presented at the AOTA Annual Conference & Expo, San Diego.

Schulz, R., & Beach, S. R. (1999). Caregiving as a risk factor for mortality: The Caregiver Health Effects Study. *JAMA, 282*, 2215–2219. http://dx.doi.org/10.1001/jama.282.23.2215

Seamon, D. (2002). Physical comminglings: Body, habit and space transformed into place. *OTJR: Occupation, Participation and Health, 22*(Suppl. 1), 425–515.

Segal, R. (2004). Family routines and rituals: A context for occupational therapy interventions.

American Journal of Occupational Therapy, 58, 499–508. http://dx.doi.org/10.5014/ajot.58.5.499

Sheikh, J. I., & Yesavage, J. A. (1986). Geriatric Depression Scale (GDS): Recent findings and development of a shorter version. In T. L. Brink (Ed.), *Clinical gerontology: A guide to assessment and intervention* (pp. 165–173). New York: Haworth Press.

Siebert, C. (2005). *Occupational therapy practice guidelines for home modifications*. Bethesda, MD: AOTA Press.

Siebert, C. (2008). Occupational patterns: Roles, habits, and routines. In S. Coppola, S. Elliott, & P. Toto (Eds.), *Strategies to advance gerontology excellence: Promoting best practice in occupational therapy* (pp. 91–107). Bethesda, MD: AOTA Press.

Stark, S. (2001). Creating disability in the home: The role of environmental barriers in the United States. *Disability and Society, 16*, 37–49. http://dx.doi.org/10.1080/713662037

Stark, S. (2004). Removing environmental barriers in the homes of older adults with disabilities improves occupational performance. *OTJR: Occupation, Participation and Health, 24*, 32–39.

Stark, S., Landsbaum, A., Palmer, J. L., Somerville, E. K., & Morris, J. C. (2009). Client-centred home modifications improve daily activity performance of older adults. *Canadian Journal of Occupational Therapy, 76*, 235–245.

Stark, S., Somerville, E., & Keglovits, M. (2013). *Tailored home modification intervention for older adults with chronic conditions*. Unpublished manual.

Stark, S. L., Somerville, E. K., & Morris, J. C. (2010). In-Home Occupational Performance Evaluation (I–HOPE). *American Journal of Occupational Therapy, 64*, 580–589. http://dx.doi.org/10.5014/ajot.2010.0z8065

Stark, S., Somerville, E., & Russell-Thomas, D. (2011). Choosing assessments for home modifications. In M. Christenson & C. Chase (Eds.), *Occupational therapy and home modifications: Promoting safety and supporting participation* (pp. 25–43). Bethesda, MD: AOTA Press.

Steinfeld, E., & Shea, S. (1993). Enabling home environments: Identifying barriers to independence. *Technology and Disability, 2,* 69–79.

Stevens, J. A., Corso, P. S., Finkelstein, E. A., & Miller, T. R. (2006). The costs of fatal and nonfatal falls among older adults. *Injury Prevention, 12,* 290–295. http://dx.doi.org/10.1136/ip.2005.011015

Tabbarah, M., Silverstein, M., & Seeman, T. (2000). A health and demographic profile of noninstitutionalized older Americans residing in environments with home modifications. *Journal of Aging and Health, 12,* 204–228. http://dx.doi.org/10.1177/089826430001200204

Taylor, R. R., & Van Puymbroeck, L. (2013). Therapeutic use of self: Applying the intentional relationship model in group therapy. In J. C. O'Brien & J. W. Solomon (Eds.), *Occupational analysis and group process* (pp. 36–52). St. Louis: Elsevier.

Tinetti, M. E., Baker, D. I., Gottschalk, M., Williams, C. S., Pollack, D., Garrett, P., . . . Acampora, D. (1999). Home-based multicomponent rehabilitation program for older persons after hip fracture: A randomized trial. *Archives of Physical Medicine and Rehabilitation, 80,* 916–922. http://dx.doi.org/10.1016/S0003-9993(99)90083-7

Tomita, M. R., Mann, W. C., Stanton, K., Tomita, A. D., & Sundar, V. (2007). Use of currently available smart home technology by frail elders: Process and outcomes. *Topics in Geriatric Rehabilitation, 23,* 24–34.

Townsend, E., & Wilcock, A. A. (2004). Occupational justice and client-centred practice: A dialogue in progress. *Canadian Journal of Occupational Therapy, 71,* 75–87. http://dx.doi.org/10.1177/000841740407100203

Trombly, C. A. (1995). Occupation: Purposefulness and meaningfulness as therapeutic mechanisms [Eleanor Clarke Slagle Lecture]. *American Journal of Occupational Therapy, 49,* 960–972. http://dx.doi.org/10.5014/ajot.49.10.960

Tuan, Y.-F. (1977). *Space and place: The perspective of experience.* Minneapolis: University of Minnesota Press.

U.S. Preventive Services Task Force. (2012). *Grade definitions.* Retrieved from http://www.uspreventiveservicestaskforce.org/uspstf/grades.htm

van Haastregt, J. C., Diederiks, J. P., van Rossum, E., de Witte, L. P., Voorhoeve, P. M., & Crebolder, H. F. (2000). Effects of a programme of multifactorial home visits on falls and mobility impairments in elderly people at risk: Randomised controlled trial. *BMJ, 321,* 994–998. http://dx.doi.org/10.1136/bmj.321.7267.994

Velligan, D. I., Diamond, P. M., Maples, N. J., Mintz, J., Li, X., Glahn, D. C., & Miller, A. L. (2008). Comparing the efficacy of interventions that use environmental supports to improve outcomes in patients with schizophrenia. *Schizophrenia Research, 102,* 312–319.

Velligan, D. I., Diamond, P., Mueller, J., Li, X., Maples, N., Wang, M., & Miller, A. L. (2009). The short-term impact of generic versus individualized environmental supports on functional outcomes and target behaviors in schizophrenia. *Psychiatry Research, 168,* 94–101. http://dx.doi.org/10.1016/j.psychres.2008.03.016

Ware, J. E., Jr., & Sherbourne, C. D. (1992). The MOS 36-item Short-Form Health Survey (SF–36): I. Conceptual framework and item selection. *Medical Care, 30,* 473–483.

Warren, M. (1998). *Brain Injury Visual Assessment Battery for Adults*. Lenexa, KS: visABILITIES Rehab Services.

Watson, D. E., & Llorens, L. A. (1997). *Task analysis: An occupational performance approach.* Bethesda, MD: American Occupational Therapy Association.

Watson, D. E., & Wilson, S. A. (2003). *Task analysis: An individual and population approach* (2nd ed.). Bethesda, MD: AOTA Press.

Whelan, L. R. (2014). Assessing abilities and capacities: Range of motion, strength, and endurance in occupational therapy for physical dysfunction. In. M. Vining Radomski & C. A. Trombly Latham (Eds.), *Occupational therapy for physical dysfunction* (7th ed., pp.144–241). Baltimore: Lippincott Williams & Wilkins.

Wilson, D. J., Mitchell, J. M., Kemp, B. J., Adkins, R. H., & Mann, W. (2009). Effects of assistive technology on functional decline in people aging with a disability. *Assistive Technology, 21,* 208–217. http://dx.doi.org/10.1080/10400430903246068

World Health Organization. (2001). *International classification of functioning, disability and health*. Geneva: Author.

Yardley, L., Beyer, N., Hauer, K., Kempen, G., Piot-Ziegler, C., & Todd, C. (2005). Development and initial validation of the Falls Efficacy Scale-International (FES–I). *Age and Ageing, 34,* 614–619. http://dx.doi.org/10.1093/ageing/afi196

Subject Index

Note. Page numbers in *italics* indicate figures, and tables.

client factors, 17–18, *18*
evaluation, 11–12, *13*
occupational performance, 14, 34–35
occupational profile, 12–14
of occupational therapy, 3–5, *4*
performance patterns, 18–20
performance skills, 16–17
referrals, 11
process skills, 16–17
see also performance skills

quality of life, 35

Rebuilding Together, 40
referrals, 11, 38–39
see also process
regulation of occupational therapy practice, 60
reimbursement, 23
research
implications for, 55–56
review of, 43
search strategies, 64–65, *64*
residents, needs of, 31
rituals, 20
see also performance patterns
role competence, 37
roles, 19–20
see also performance patterns
routines, 19
see also performance patterns

Safety Assessment of Function and the
Environment for Rehabilitation–Health
Outcome Measurement Evaluation, Version 3
(SAFER), *13*, 16, 40

safety audits, 23–24
schizophrenia, 51
search strategies, 64–65, *64*
service delivery contexts, 8
single-component interventions, 45
smart homes (SHs), *87*
social demands, 29
see also intervention planning
social environment, 22
see also contexts
social interaction skills, 17
see also performance skills
space demands, 28–29
see also intervention planning
Stepping On, *69*
strategies, behavioral, 26
see also intervention

task analysis, 28
see also intervention planning
task lighting, *68*
team approach, 23, 26
see also intervention
temporal context, 22
see also contexts
theoretical approaches, 27–28

virtual environment, 22
see also contexts

well-being, 37
wellness, 35
Westmead Home Safety Assessment, *13*

Citation Index

Note. Page numbers in *italics* indicate tables.

Westbury, C., 44, 45, *70*
Whelan, L. R., *18*
Wilcock, A. A., 37
Williams, C. S., 44, 48, 50, *87*
Wilson, D. J., 48, 50, 51, 53, *90*
Wilson, S. A., 17
Winter, L., 7, *13*, 48, 51, 52, *66*, *72*, *74*, *75*

Wittstein, I. S., 51
Wolf, M., 43
Wolf, S. L., 44, 45, 46, *72*

Yardley, L., 47
Yesavage, J. A., *18*
Youngstrom, M. J., 25